Dear Governor:

About the State of Reform

Dear Governor:

About the State of Reform

Edited by D.J. Wilson

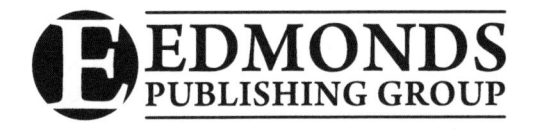

EDMONDS PUBLISHING GROUP

Lynnwood, Washington

Published by
Edmonds Publishing Group
3500 188th St. Suite 590
Lynnwood, WA 98037
www.stateofreform.com

The Edmonds Publishing Group is an independent publisher located in Lynnwood, Washington. Our mission is to foster dialogue among and between civic leaders in the hopes of advancing public policy that will best serve the common good.

Copyright © 2012 Edmonds Publishing Group

All rights reserved. No part of this book may be reproduced in any manner without the prior written permission of the publisher, except as provided by USA copyright law.

ISBN: 978-0-9881836-0-5
Library of Congress Control Number: 2012946438

Editor: D.J. Wilson

Printed and bound in the United States of America.

Table of Contents

Introduction

D.J. Wilson 3
>   *Editor*
>   Dear Governor: About the State of Reform

Five Minutes with the Governor

Alan Yordy 15
>   *President and Chief Mission Officer*
>   PeaceHealth

John Franson 21
>   *Family Practice Physician*
>   Lakeview Medical Clinic

Lon G. Wilson 17
>   *President*
>   The Wilson Agency

Stephen Rose 35
>   *Partner*
>   Garvey Schubert Barer

Roger Stark 41
   Health Care Policy Analyst
   Washington Policy Center

Gubby Barlow 47
   President and Chief Executive Officer
   Premera Blue Cross

David Rolf 55
   President
   SEIU Healthcare 775NW

Scott Kreiling 61
   President
   Regence BlueShield of Idaho

Aaron Katz 67
   Principal Lecturer of Health Services and Global Health
   University of Washington

Scott Armstrong 71
   President and Chief Executive Officer
   Group Health Cooperative

DONALD FISHER 77
    Chief Executive Officer
    American Medical Group Association

TOM FRITZ 85
    Chief Executive Officer
    INHS

TIMOTHY BROWN 91
    Executive Director
    Terry Reilly

MAGGIE BENNINGTON-DAVIS.. 95
    Chief Medical and Operating Officer
    Cascadia Behavioral Healthcare

JOHN HOOPES 101
    Chief Executive Officer
    Caribou Memorial Hospital

MELINDA MULLER 107
    Clinical Vice President, Primary Care
    Legacy Medical Group
    Legacy Health

MARILYN KASMAR 111
    Former Chief Executive Officer
    Alaska Primary Care Association

RICHARD H. COOPER 117
    Chief Executive Officer
    The Everett Clinic

ACKNOWLEDGEMENTS 125

ABOUT THE EDITOR 127

ABOUT THE STATE OF REFORM 129

Introduction

DEAR GOVERNOR:

ALASKA
IDAHO
OREGON
WASHINGTON

D.J. WILSON

Editor
Dear Governor: About the State of Reform

If you had five minutes with the Governor to talk healthcare, what would you say?

That's the question we asked 18 healthcare, business, civic and legal executives from across four states: Washington, Oregon, Idaho and Alaska.

The response, collected here in "Dear Governor: About the State of Reform," offers readers a sophisticated level of discussion and analysis of healthcare policy in the northwest.

The four states are as diverse as any in the country, ranging from fully engaged in reform to fully oppositional. It reminds me that the old adage about physician offices rings true in the states; if you've seen one state address the challenges of healthcare, you've seen only one state.

> *DJ Wilson is President of Wilson Strategic Communications, one of the region's leading healthcare strategy and public affairs firms. He also hosts the State of Reform Health Policy Conferences held annually in Washington, Alaska, Idaho, and Oregon.*

DEAR GOVERNOR:

In other words, the reforms implemented in one state are only an uneasy fit for the state just across the border.

That said, there is tremendous value in sharing the approach and considerations otherwise disparate healthcare players are each taking in today's anxious environment. Indeed, the thinking and discussions in advance of the actual decisions may be more insightful than the actual decisions themselves, whether there is an exact fit across silos or not.

Knowing how these leaders think about the challenges we all face – increasing cost, sporadic quality, limited access – is of tremendous value.

Sharing this knowledge is the purpose of this book – to seed thoughtful discussion of one of the most challenging topics in public policy, in society, and in our democracy today: healthcare.

In addition to our conferences and our online healthcare news site, www.stateofreform.com, this book hopes to foster a dialogue among different and credible viewpoints interested in solutions and collaboration.

*   *   *

These are interesting times to be in healthcare.

The passage of the Affordable Care Act represents the most transformational piece of healthcare legislation in almost a half century. It reshapes the insurance marketplace for consumers, provides funds to expand coverage, and supports innovations in payment reform and care coordination that have tremendous potential.

The law has also helped create more uncertainty, anxiety, and nervousness in the healthcare marketplace than has existed at any other time in recent memory.

In fact, there has not been this much change happening in healthcare since the advent of Medicare and Medicaid under Lyndon Johnson's "Great Society."

States like Oregon are fully embracing the challenge. Governor John Kitzhaber grabbed headlines with the development of care coordination organizations, and the extensive funding – $1.9 billion[1] – offered by CMS to frontload the transformation there.

Washington State has been awarded more federal grant money – $151.8 million[2] – to implement a health benefit exchange than any state in the country. The role of the exchange, while still developing, has the potential to reshape the entire consumer marketplace, shifting insurance purchasing from the hands of employers directly to employees.

In Idaho and Alaska, a cautious approach to the Affordable Care Act has not dampened the fundamental belief at all levels of the market and government that changing the healthcare system continues to be vital to moving the economy forward.

The amount of change in healthcare today is matched only by the

---

[1] Kiff, Sarah. "White House makes $1.9 billion bet: Oregon can fix health care." Washington Post. http://www.washingtonpost.com/blogs/ezra-klein/post/white-house-makes-19-billion-bet-oregon-can-fix-health-care/2012/05/04/gIQAz3AB1T_blog.html.

[2] Total Health Insurance Exchange Grants, 2012. Kaiser Family Foundation. http://statehealthfacts.kff.org/comparetable.jsp?ind=964&cat=17.

DEAR GOVERNOR:

pace of change. Executives at Group Health Cooperative, a consumer-governed, nonprofit health care system in Seattle, repeat the mantra "Grow confident making decisions amidst the chaos." Those are wise words for us all.

This is why we've put together this book. In times of anxiety and uncertainty, collaboration among colleagues with like-minded values and interests can become a key to success.

For all of the time we spend thinking about competitive advantages or highlighting the divergence of our interests, at the end of the day, both as citizens and as leaders, the healthcare community will likely all agree on the importance of moving beyond the status quo.

Change is needed, and for that, collaboration is required.

* * *

These are interesting times to be in this economy.

Since our last book in 2008, the "Great Recession" has struck America like a sledgehammer – hitting all states, but states like Oregon and Washington harder than many others.

Across the board in the northwest, the number of unemployed workers continues to be higher in 2012 than at the start of the recession.

In Alaska and Idaho, the numbers of unemployed workers are up 16% and 8%, respectively, today over four years ago.

	AK June 2008	AK June 2012	ID June 2008	ID June 2012
Labor Force	356,596	367,745	751,061	781,869
Employment	333,643	341,079	695,587	721,935
Unemployment	22,953	26,666	55,474	59,934
Unemployment Rate	6.4	7.3	7.4	7.7

In Washington and Oregon, the numbers of unemployed workers in 2012 compared to 2008 are dramatically worse: up 61% and 45%, respectively.

Moreover, in those two states, the total number of employed workers statewide in June 2012 continues to be less than the number of employed workers in June, 2008.[3] This has all happened while the general population has increased in both states.

In an economy where one's access to health insurance has historically been tied to one's access to a full time job, these numbers alone are more than simply unsettling.

But they don't tell the whole story.

When one reviews the number of underemployed in the area – those defined as unemployed, workers employed part-time for economic reasons, and those only marginally attached to the labor force – the four state northwest economy gets even more troubling.

---

[3] Bureau of Labor Statistics. US Department of Labor. www.bls.gov.

DEAR GOVERNOR:

	WA June 2008	WA June 2012	OR June 2008	OR June 2012
Labor Force	3,463,276	3,525,177	1,952,178	1,987,542
Employment	3,282,178	3,231,932	1,835,409	1,818,673
Unemployment	181,098	293,245	116,769	168,869
Unemployment Rate	5.2	8.3	6.0	8.5

Because this measure of underemployment counts part-time and marginally employed workers, it's likely that this is a more accurate measure of workers looking for full time work – with the medical benefits which often accompany full time work.

However, data on unemployment can tend to be abstract. An even more accurate indicator of how the economy is performing, and consequently how secure one might feel with one's employer based insurance coverage, can be found in how "close to home" the recession has been felt. In other words, has the economy impacted you and your health insurance?

Here are some numbers that help tell that part of the story.

In 2010, 58.7 million Americans had no health insurance for at least part of the previous 12-month period. That number accounts for roughly one in six of all Americans.

That number is distorted, however, by the inclusion of seniors on Medicare and low income folks eligible for Medicaid.

If we look at just middle income families ($43,000 to $65,000) for a family of four at just the middle years of their lives

ABOUT THE STATE OF REFORM

2011 Annual Rates of Unemployment by State According to BLS [4]	US	WA	OR	AK	ID
Unemployment[5]	8.9	9.4	9.4	7.6	8.7
Underemployment rate[6]	15.9	17.8	17.5	13.5	16.1

(18-64 years old), 1 in 3 individuals went without health insurance at some point during the previous 12-month period.[7]

One in three working age, middle income adults had no health insurance at some point in the previous 12 months.

That is the kind of number that means health care insecurity, brought on by a challenging economy, is no longer an abstract notion for many middle income families.

This is why we've put together this book. Putting our healthcare system on a more fundamentally sound path moving forward is something we can all agree is a priority.

---

[4] Table 2. "Alternative Measures of Labor Underutilization, California – 2011." Bureau of Labor Statistics. http://www.bls.gov/ro9/altca.htm#table2

[5] This number, the U-3 unemployment number, is defined as all jobless persons who are available to take a job and have actively sought work in the past four weeks as a percentage of the total labor force.

[6] This number, the U-6 unemployment number, includes the unemployed, workers employed part-time for economic reasons, and the marginally attached to the labor force.

[7] "Vital Signs: Health Insurance Coverage and Health Care Utilization --- United States, 2006--2009 and January--March 2010." Centers for Disease Control and Prevention. www.cdc.gov.

This conversation matters – to us all.

* * *

These are interesting times to be a citizen.

Respectful civic dialogue about the primary issues of the day is an endangered species. Today, pundits make a living on cable TV, talk radio and online by using hyperbole and overgeneralizations. They teach us that talking past one another is more important than listening to one another.

At both ends of the political spectrum, some believe that using half-truths and falsehoods to mobilize a constituency is part of the game rather than a degradation of our common social bonds.

Those social bonds – the trust we have in one another and our faith in self-government – are frayed. Never in my life have I seen as broad and as deep a sense among regular citizens that, sadly, perhaps our system of government cannot solve the problems before us.

Just as sad – to me – are the flip comments thrown around by some civic leaders and which pass for civil debate.

Words are powerful. They have meaning and shape the way we define our reality.

Terms like "death panels," statements like "kill the wealthy" and phraseology that frames the goal as conflict rather than compromise all severely undermine our ability to be successful. Here, Bill Maher is just as damaging as Rush Limbaugh.

This is why we've put together this book. By combining key thought leaders from health care in one place, this book provides a snapshot of the kind of civic discourse health care demands today.

These authors provide a window into the policy discussions and strategic deliberations happening across health care today, from the provider office to the caucus meeting room.

More importantly, they offer a thoughtful, respectful policy dialogue meritorious of the governor's attention – and ours as citizens.

* * *

It comes down to this: in a republican democracy, whether you are a Republican or a Democrat, we are all in this together.

And, now as much as ever, our attention on healthcare, the economy, and our civic discourse must be careful, constructive, and deliberate.

Five Minutes with the Governor

DEAR GOVERNOR:

ALASKA
OREGON
WASHINGTON

Alan Yordy

President and Chief Mission Officer
PeaceHealth

Dear Governor,

You are responsible for serving the same people we are. Every single resident of your state will eventually need our services – for hospitalization, immunization, or anything in between.

And that starts us off on common ground as, in order to meet the needs of the constituency we share, we strive to work together to overcome our biggest obstacle: how to reconcile the promises we've made and entitlements we've granted with the resources we have to fund those commitments.

What has the potential to divide us is our fiduciary responsibility – yours to state government, and mine to the nonprofit organization I lead. Neither one of us can fulfill our sacred obligation if health care providers can no longer maintain creditworthiness

> *Alan began his health care career in PeaceHealth's Oregon Region in the early 1980s. In 1990 he left to become CEO of Mid-Valley Healthcare, and in 1997 he co-founded Samaritan Health Services in Oregon's Linn and Benton counties. Alan returned to PeaceHealth in 1999 as Chief Executive Officer of the Oregon Region. He assumed his current system-wide leadership role in 2005.*

and critical access to capital that has allowed us to create one of the world's best health care systems.

And this brings us back to the challenge of reconciling available funding with the promise of a health benefits package that is sustainable.

Health care leaders know how to achieve the so-called "triple aim" of health care – to improve population health, enhance the patient experience and control costs – but we can't do it if the majority of our patients – those who are government-sponsored or who are uninsured altogether – rely on subsidization by the private sector.

Under current law, the government is poised to expand Medicaid to cover more low-income and uninsured – a population we all agree deserves decent health care – while paying little more than half the actual cost of delivering that care.

Receiving about 50 cents for every dollar expended is more than unaffordable; it demands that we examine the justice of promising care to one population by requiring another to fund a significant portion of the cost of that care.

It's tempting to let other issues, such as public employee benefits or private-sector pay, distract us from the fundamental problem at hand: the cost of health care is more than we want to pay, largely because health care can do things it couldn't do before.

Clearly, we can find greater efficiencies in care delivery. One recent study suggested that we could reduce the cost of care by 10 to 15 percent for the primary Medicaid population.

But the fact remains that, as much as we can criticize our outcomes when compared to other countries, we live longer and do more than we used to thanks to medical advances that largely originated in the United States.

The Pacific Northwest is home to a greater number of uninsured than most other states. According to one study, the uninsured rate ranges from 7th highest in the country in Alaska to 26th in Washington, with Idaho and Oregon falling between them at 14th and 20th respectively.

Clearly, this isn't good.

We are also home to the highest percentage of Catholic hospitals in the country. Coupled with other nonprofit hospital systems that dominate in our region, we have a unique opportunity to partner with the state in service to the public.

That is an advantage which I hope we recognize and use.

I believe the conversations about how to address the health care funding problem will be far more productive and successful if we can acknowledge some perhaps unpopular realities:

- Prevention may cost us more than we are paying today in the short run. It is the right thing to do, and in many individual cases prevention is less expensive than treatment of disease. But we can't expect our state and national health care bill to decline simply because we've added preventive services; in fact, some experts predict the opposite will happen.

- Obesity is growing rapidly in the United States. Roughly one-third of all adults are now considered more than 120 percent of their ideal body mass. This trend is highly correlated to many other chronic diseases and will require public policy debate and intervention if it is to be reversed.

- Health care will continue to become more costly as we continue to discover new, more effective treatments. Unless we choose to halt progress and adopt an approach similar to other developed countries, which limit access to expensive technology, we must factor the cost of discovery into our calculations.

- Most Americans have access to the health care system, especially in our region with its dominance of nonprofit, mission-driven health care organizations. While patchwork in nature and unevenly organized, the system provides care to people in need regardless of their insurance status. That doesn't diminish the fact that the system is often confusing and difficult to navigate, especially for the most vulnerable among us.

- There is room for improvement at all levels – quality, service, access and cost. And great progress is being made on all fronts. Quality continues to improve at America's best hospitals. Costs per unit of care will continue to stabilize as health care systems across the Northwest become more efficient. It requires resources to implement the changes we want to see, and neither the government nor the private sector has them.

We will be successful only if we regard one another as partners, not adversaries. We must earn and keep one another's trust.

We cannot afford to fail, because too much is at stake for the organizations we represent and the people we serve.

Neither one of us, alone, has the solution. Together, I pray we can find it.

Respectfully yours,

Alan Yordy

DEAR GOVERNOR:

IDAHO

JOHN FRANSON

Family Practice Physician
Lakeview Medical Clinic

Dear Governor,

As a family physician in rural Idaho, I've often thought about the health of my community and how care could be improved.

Malpractice Reform

As you know, potential medical lawsuits in Idaho are first reviewed by panels of medical professionals. When they are considered legitimate they proceed to trial. Otherwise they are dismissed as frivolous. This screening process saves time and money.

Idaho has also set a limit on the amount that can be awarded for "pain and suffering," a real thing some patients experience but one that is both nebulous and fraught with emotion. This cap

> Dr. John Franson has practiced medicine in Soda Springs for 10 years. He works a small farm with draft horses and raises a few cows, apples and colorful potatoes.

ensures that jurors retain some measure of fiscal sanity in their deliberations. Because malpractice insurance companies, hospitals, and physicians pass costs on to patients, tort reform lowers everyone's expenses.

This is an area in which Idaho has done well. Other governors may find our experience instructive.

Medicaid Drug Contracts

An obscure feature of Idaho Medicaid is a twisted financial incentive to have patients on particular drugs, due to relationships with certain favored drug companies.

Sometimes I can prescribe a cheaper substitute but Medicaid refuses to cover it because they get a financial kickback when another drug is chosen.

As a dramatic but true example, just this month Medicaid insisted one of my patients receive a $14,000 drug (yes, fourteen thousand dollars confirmed with pharmacy) when an equivalent substitute was available for $100.

When I explained this to the patient she saw through it and insisted on paying $100 out of pocket, saying taxpayers shouldn't be gouged. True rural integrity. With another patient the price differential was $1668 per month versus $209, which adds up since that patient has remained on the drug for over 60 months now.

Co-Payments For All

Although Medicaid helps those of limited means obtain health care, we see abuse of the system. Recently Medicaid patients have been asked to pay $3.65 for each office visit. This is a step in the right direction.

It might be wise to require a copayment for emergency room visits and medication refills as well. The point is not to collect a lot of money, but to encourage appreciation and wise use of resources.

This should apply not just to Medicaid patients but those insured through the VA, Indian Health Services, Armed Forces, Workers Compensation and all other forms of health insurance that may be paying 100%.

Free rides are an illusion and in the end they often create monsters.

Electronic Medical Records

Although electronic record systems have certain niches, especially in big systems like the VA, they are not a panacea. We need to quit pretending these systems will solve the issue of costs.

Nor do they improve the quality of health care. They are expensive and cumbersome. And with over 100 products currently jousting for market share, none of which are capable of talking to each other, we have eliminated the greatest potential benefit of the EMR, which is communication between offices and hospitals.

More expensive technology will not painlessly and effortlessly solve our health care problems. From Bush to Obama we've been suckered into this. If it sounds too good to be true, it probably is.

Specialty Physicians

Just as electronic records will not make health care more affordable, neither will training more specialists. Nonetheless, graduating specialists now outnumber new primary care physicians 9:1. Perhaps unsurprisingly, Americans have increasingly bought into the notion that they need a different physician for each body part.

This is a fragmented, expensive, and neurotic way to deliver health care. Instead, we need a new wave of broadly-trained physicians capable of treating the great majority of the medical problems they encounter. When generalists and specialists are approximately equal in number, health care has its greatest potential for good.

Farm Bill

This year the national Farm Bill is being debated and revised. Among other things, the bill specifies how subsidies are allocated to farmers. With our health in mind it's time to move beyond mere token support for healthy crops.

As long as we remain a nation of corn and soybeans kept artificially cheap by price supports, we will increasingly become a nation whose health could be much better. An apple shouldn't cost more than a Twinkie. Send a little money to the farmers who grow broccoli and blueberries.

Prescription Drugs

Don't keep trying to run the local pharmacists out of business by encouraging Medicare patients to fill their prescriptions through the mail from big warehouses halfway across the country. There are many benefits to having town pharmacists who know their patients, care about them personally, and are accountable and easily accessible.

Science

Listen to scientists with regard to chemicals like BPA, even when they don't have the money and lobbyists to compete with Big Industry. Some of these products affect people's health.

Sincerely,

Dr. John Franson

DEAR GOVERNOR:

ALASKA

LON G. WILSON

President
The Wilson Agency

Dear Governor,

There is a well known parable about six blind men who are brought to an elephant and asked to describe what he felt. The first man described the tail as a rope, the second man described its ear as a fan, the third man described its tusk as a plow, and so on it went. Each description was different, yet each man was certain he knew the right answer.

Each was partly right and all were wrong. In the end, all they could do was argue.

Our health care system is much like the elephant and the stakeholders (hospitals, doctors, insurance carriers, patients, employers, and the government) much like the blind men. Each stakeholder sees their part so clearly they make suggestions, changes

Lon G. Wilson is President of The Wilson Agency, a full service strategic employee benefits consulting firm, helping Alaskan businesses to develop an organized approach to complex employee initiatives.

and accusations from that vantage point. Just like the blind men, each is partly right but none has the answer, especially if he's too invested in his own position to hear other viewpoints.

The biggest problem with our health care system is that it is expensive. Moreover, like much of what we buy as Alaskans, it costs even more here because of where we live. Consider the following data compiled by the Alaska Health Care Commission in their 2011 Annual Report:

- Health care spending has risen 40% since 2005, totaling $7.5 billion in 2010.

- On its current trajectory, health care spending in Alaska will nearly double, up to $14 billion in 2020. For comparison, the wellhead value of oil produced in Alaska is only expected to rise 13% over the same time period (from $16.4 billion in 2010 to $18.6 billion in 2020).

- The cost of medical care has been rising three times faster than inflation in Anchorage since 1982.[1]

The Commission named a number of factors that are familiar to us as Alaskans that drive prices up: "higher operating costs for providers resulting from a higher cost of living, more costly employee benefits, transportation and shipping costs, fuel prices, and workforce shortages."

Undoubtedly, our unique geography and economics creates an environment that pushes prices up. In fact, Alaska has the

---

[1] Alaska Health Care Commission 2011 Annual Report, http://www.hss.state.ak.us/healthcommission/docs/2011_report%201-15-12_final.pdf, Executive Summary, page IV.

"highest average annual cost for employee health insurance in the nation" ($11,926 per employee)[2]. As costs rise every year, fewer employers offer health insurance and those that do end up offering smaller and smaller benefit packages.

While it's true that living here is expensive, we should not accept the exploding cost of medical care that is driving the price of health insurance and hurting both businesses and individual citizens.

Our elephant is hemorrhaging and we need to find the cause so that we can apply pressure to stop the bleeding. This dramatic increase in costs is clearly not sustainable and the business community regularly tells me this is not acceptable and something must be done. The growing amount of money spent by employers on health care coverage is money that isn't being spent on hiring new employees, giving employee raises thus increasing their spending power or investing in businesses to help them grow. The growth of businesses in Alaska is something we all need to care about.

In order to contain costs, it's important to know what drives the cost of health care and understand why it is so much more expensive in Alaska. Fortunately, we can again look to the Alaska Health Care Commission and their recent report that put a fine point on the critical issue of rising costs.

In their report, the Commission stated that: "[c]ommercial insurance premiums are primarily a factor of utilization and price for health care services" and that "[u]tilization of health care ser-

---

[2] United Benefit Advisors 2011 Health Plan Survey.

vices in Alaska is roughly in line with comparison states, and is lower than nationwide average."[3]

If insurance premiums are established primarily through utilization and price for services, and Alaska's utilization is at or below average, then one can easily conclude that the price for services must be the primary driver of the cost of health insurance. In fact, the Commission substantiates this, stating, "[h]igher prices [in Alaska] are also due to high physician pricing power compared to other states..."[4]

Demonstrated examples included:

- Reimbursement for physician services in Alaska is 60% higher than in comparison states for all payers based on a weighted average; and 69% higher for commercial (private insurance) payers.

- The difference in reimbursement for physician services varies significantly depending on the specialty. Pediatricians in Alaska are reimbursed at rates 43% higher on average than pediatricians in the comparison states, and cardiologists in Alaska are reimbursed at rates 83% higher than cardiologists in the comparison states.

- Commercial reimbursement for private sector hospital services is 37% higher in Alaska than in the comparison states. Medicare fees paid for private sector hospital services are

---

[3] Alaska Health Care Commission 2011 Annual Report, http://www.hss.state.ak.us/healthcommission/docs/2011_report%201-15-12_final.pdf, page 12.

[4] Ibid, page iv.

36% higher in Alaska than in the comparison states. [5]

Moreover, the Commission also found "[p]hysician discounts are low in Alaska, an indication that physicians in Alaska have more market power relative to pricing." I certainly don't want to unfairly target one particular stakeholder in our system, but it does beg the question…why?

In the report, the Commission answered that question quite clearly: "There are state laws and regulations in place that influence the market in such a way as to drive prices higher for the consumer." [6] Beyond the general lack of competition, the report is referring to two particular pieces of legislation.

First is a state regulation requiring health insurers pay "the 80th percentile of billed charges." However, if a provider has a certain market share, which many of them do, providers can generally charge prices in a way that ensures they will be paid what they want. In plainer English: there is no incentive for providers to contract with health insurers when they get paid for their full billed charges, no matter how high, resulting in charges that are not affordable for consumers, employees and employers.

Second is a state law that requires insurers to "reimburse non-contracted providers directly." [7] So, even if you pay the provider upfront for a service and submit the claim, the insurance company is required by state regulations to send the check to the provider. In contrast, insurers in other states send a check to the

---

[5] Ibid, page 13.

[6] Ibid, page 13.

[7] Ibid.

insured, allowing the individual to settle the bill directly with the out-of-network provider. Again, providers lack incentive to contract with insurance companies and since they have no need to negotiate their price, it ultimately drives up costs for consumers.

Think about it this way: when you purchase insurance, you're not only protecting yourself from a major potential financial liability in the event of serious injury or illness, you're also hiring the insurance company to negotiate the best possible deal on your behalf. Yet, the way things currently work in Alaska, your insurer is essentially forced to negotiate with one hand behind their back.

It's no wonder an independent study prepared for the Alaska Health Care Commission found provider reimbursement in Alaska 69% higher than in comparison states. [8] That fact explains a lot about why our premiums are so high.

It also makes clear that the Legislature could do everyone who pays for health care coverage a favor by addressing this state regulation on "billed charges" and the state law on payments to doctors.

Obviously, there are other factors contributing to Alaska's large health care costs. Our population is aging and growing more obese. [9] At the same time, amazing new medical technology also comes at a price. Cost shifting from public payers that pay less force commercial payers to pick up more of the tab. Those are tougher issues to address, even if they still merit our attention.

---

[8] Ibid., Appendix B, Part 3, "Drivers of Health Care Costs in Alaska and Comparison States," Milliman, Inc., http://www.hss.state.ak.us/healthcommission/docs/drivers_healthcare_costs.pdf, Executive Summary, page 2.

[9] Center for Health Data and Statistics http://www.hss.state.ak.us/dph/infocenter/

But, it's clear from the Alaska Health Care Commission's findings that there are some simpler and more achievable steps our Legislature could take right now to reduce government regulations in the health insurance marketplace and begin reducing health care costs for Alaskans. It's just good business.

After all, how does one "eat" an elephant? One bite at a time, according to my young son. But unless we want to dismantle our health care system, we need to figure out how to make it move and work for us instead of blindly hacking away in the hopes that a solution comes with dinner.

Sincerely,

Lon G. Wilson

DEAR GOVERNOR:

ALASKA
OREGON
WASHINGTON

STEPHEN ROSE

Partner
Garvey Schubert Barer

Dear Governor,

I believe that everyone – healthcare providers, the Alaska State Medicaid program, the federal Medicare program, insurance companies, and other third party payers – agrees that fraud, abuse, and waste within the healthcare delivery system must be eliminated. To that end, conducting audits of health care providers makes sense.

However now it seems that an endless procession of audits has been launched. Keeping in mind that each of these audits requires the diversion of scarce healthcare resources to respond to them, I have to wonder whether all of these audits are necessary.

A recent federal Government Accountability Office (GAO) report concluded that at least one federal Medicaid audit program cost five times more to administer than was being recovered. [1]

Stephen Rose is Chair of the Health Care Law Section of Garvey Schubert Barer. He has more than 25 years of experience representing clients in the healthcare industry responding to government audits. He has also worked for the Washington State Medical Association preparing and presenting educational materials for their membership on both the HIPAA Privacy Rule, Security Standard and HITECH Act.

DEAR GOVERNOR:

In other words, for every $5.00 of taxpayer money spent $1.00 was recovered as an improper Medicaid overpayment.

The cost of administration is only part of the story as the total cost number does not include the tens of millions of dollars that the health care providers had to incur in order to respond to the government audit.

Very few people know what is required to respond to a government audit.

The typical audit starts with the auditors asking for information. The provider then has to assign employees to gather that information for the auditors. The information is then supplied in either electronic or hard copy. The auditors then process the information.

After the information is processed, the auditors (usually) request clarifications and interviews of the health care providers employees. Eventually the auditors provide a written report.

Once the report is provided, the health care provider has to review and understand the report which oftentimes requires the hiring of accountants and reimbursement specialists. If the provider disagrees with the results, appeals are usually allowed but often require that an attorney be hired.

Appeals begin at the administrative agency level, then to the lower courts, and then to the state Supreme Court. The appeals can take over a year and can cost many tens of thousands of dollars.

---

[1] GAO-12-814T, National Medicaid Audit Program Report, June 14, 2012. Report notes that the CMS Medicaid Integrity Group (MIG) spent over $100 million paid to auditors who found $20 million in overpayments.

The State of Alaska is about to launch its Medicaid Recovery Audit Contractor program along with its other Medicaid audit programs already in place. I wonder whether anyone has ever performed a cost-benefit analysis of the current Medicaid audit program. Are there redundancies and overlapping between the various audits that cost healthcare providers time and money, but which are not really cost effective?

As you are aware, there are numerous federal and state payment audits of healthcare providers. The following are just a few of the many:

- RAC Audits—Medicare Recovery Audit Contractors
- ZPIC Audits—Zone Program Integrity Contractor Audits
- PERM Audits—Payment Error Rate Measurement Audits
- CERT Audits—Comprehensive Error Rate Testing Audits
- SURS Audits—Surveillance and Utilization Review Audits
- HPMP Audits—Hospital Payment Monitoring Program Audits
- FI Billing Audits—Fiscal Intermediary Billing Audits
- POR Audits—Provider On Review Audits

This list is not exhaustive and includes only some of the payment audits. It does not include the myriad of non-payment audits such as HIPAA Audits or quality control audits.

In reviewing the above list, at least seven of audits seek to iden-

DEAR GOVERNOR:

tify whether an incorrect amount has been paid to the provider or whether a payment was made for non-covered services: RAC, ZPIC, PERM, CERT, HPMP, FI, and the current Alaska Medicaid Provider Audits.

Six of the above audits target whether there is a "medical necessity" for the healthcare services provided: RAC, ZPIC, PERM, HPMP, FI, and the current Alaska Medicaid Provider Audits.

Does a healthcare provider really need to be audited seven different times in seven different ways to determine whether they were paid for a non-covered service?

Or audited six times to determine whether the services provided were "medically necessary?"

In spite of all of the audits noted above, the federal government has now mandated that state Medicaid programs conduct Medicaid RAC Audits. The State of Alaska will soon begin its Medicaid RAC Audits.

Has anyone looked at whether these new audits will be redundant of existing audits? Has anyone determined whether there are any areas of overlap? Has the new Medicaid RAC audit been designed in a way so that it will not repeat audit areas already covered by the existing Alaska Medicaid Audits?

Or, looked at a little differently, has the State of Alaska asked whether all or part of the current Alaska Medicaid Audit program can be dispensed with as being duplicative of the new Alaska Medicaid RAC Audit program?

As I stated, I do not believe any legitimate healthcare provider disagrees with the quest to end fraud, waste, and abuse in the health care delivery system.

However, at a time when the government, both state and federal, is demanding that health care providers become more efficient and eliminate unnecessary costs, shouldn't the government demand the same of itself?

Sincerely,

Stephen Rose

DEAR GOVERNOR:

WASHINGTON

ROGER STARK

Health Care Policy Analyst
Washington Policy Center

Dear Governor,

The fundamental problem with the health care system in this country is its ever-rising cost. We spent 17% of our gross domestic product, or nearly $2.5 trillion, on health care in 2011. Most policy proposals attempt to control these expenses by imposing more top-down regulations, "better" medicine, and ultimately, a government-managed system.

Costs will continue to increase as long as each of us believes someone else will pay for our health care. Whether it is a government agency or an employer, a third party is now paying over 87% of health care costs, even as individual co-pays and deductibles are increasing. As long as we think someone else is picking up the tab, demand and utilization will far outstrip supply. This is an immutable economic law and the third-party payer problem

> Dr. Roger Stark is a retired cardiac surgeon and a health care policy analyst with Washington Policy Center, a non-partisan independent policy research organization in Washington state. He is the author of the newly released book "The Patient Centered Solution; Our Health Care Crisis, How It Happened, and How We Can Fix It."

must be solved before any reform will work.

Only when people can direct their own medical spending through a free market will costs become transparent and likewise come under control. Health services are like any other economic activity, and because of their highly complex nature, they can only be managed through the unregulated interaction of providers and patients.

Unless patients can control their own health care dollars, any reform is doomed to fail, and will lead to over utilization, uncontrolled spending, and ultimately to some form of medical rationing.

At present, there are five solutions to our current health care problem:

Change the Tax Code

Congress should change the federal tax code and allow individuals to deduct their health expenses just as businesses and privately insured self-employed individuals do now.

This would give employees the freedom to purchase their own insurance and would allow employers to crease their overhead and offer higher wages.

Individual insurance coverage, not tied to employment, would also allow people to keep their health care coverage as they move from job to job, and from state to state.

Why should an employer provide health benefits in the first place? Except for retirement plans, there are very few other needs in life, like food and housing, that are provided by employers.

Changing the tax code is obviously a federal issue, but elected state officials should lead this debate.

Eliminate Some State Mandates

Mandates set by state policymakers now restrict patient choice in the purchase of individual health insurance. Instead of offering people a range of choices, mandates require all individual plans to provide the same benefits and increase costs for everyone.

For example, why should a twenty-five-year-old, single man be forced to pay for obstetrical coverage?

Mandates are the classic example of politically-powerful lobby groups inducing policymakers to include their services in every insurance policy. Washington state has 58 mandates, whereas Idaho has only 17.

A reasonable first step would be to allow interstate commerce in health insurance. People could then purchase any approved insurance plan from any company in any state. Literally overnight, consumers would have a huge increase in personal choices and the health insurance market would become much more competitive.

Reform Medicaid

Medicaid, the program for poor families, is in an unsustainable financial condition.

We must care for the poor, but giving them mandated, unlimited, first-dollar coverage is both financially and ethically unsound. A voucher system allowing personal choice and a financial reward for dollars saved would be an excellent start to solving Medicaid's problems.

States should also receive Medicaid waivers and block grants from the federal government. States could budget more efficiently with a fixed yearly amount of money rather than the open-ended entitlement of the current Medicaid program. They could also design their own innovative programs without being stopped by the federal government.

States should be allowed to return to the original income requirement of 133 percent of the federal poverty level for their Medicaid recipients, instead of the 250 to 300 percent they now use.

Enact Tort Reform

Nearly 20 percent of our health care budget is spent on the legal system through attorneys' fees, court costs, malpractice insurance premiums, and most importantly, defensive medicine. Medical outcomes in the U.S. are no worse, and in many ways much better, than in other countries, yet our legal system burdens doctors and hospitals much more than the legal systems in other countries.

Meaningful caps on non-economic damages offer the main solution to our current legal awards lottery.

Make Health "Insurance" True Risk Management Insurance

We also need to fundamentally change how we view health insurance. Instead of "insurance" paying for every health-related activity, it needs to work like other forms of risk management insurance such as car and home owners insurance.

Just as no one uses insurance to pay for gas or to mow the lawn, we need to get away from the idea of health insurance covering all minor health-related events. True indemnity insurance should be there for unexpected catastrophes and emergencies. Day-to-day health expenses should be paid out of pocket.

An effective mechanism to do this today is a health savings account (HSA). These are being used by an increasing number of Americans. HSAs require a person or family to purchase a high-deductable catastrophic policy, but allow a tax-advantaged savings account for day-to-day medical purchases. Savings can be rolled over from year to year and are portable from one job to another.

Conclusion

These five solutions offer the best way out of our health care crisis. Given control of their health care dollars, patients, acting as health care consumers, would demand more transparency in pricing and, just as happens in other areas of life, would force competition, improve quality and service, and drive costs down.

Sincerely,

Dr. Roger Stark, MD, FACS

DEAR GOVERNOR:

ALASKA
OREGON
WASHINGTON

GUBBY BARLOW

President and Chief Executive Officer
Premera Blue Cross

Dear Governor,

We are facing an unprecedented set of healthcare challenges in our region and across the nation – challenges that transcend the debate over the future of the Affordable Care Act.

Yes, the law dramatically changes how health insurance works in America. In the long term, the ACA will fundamentally change how consumers buy coverage and how employers offer benefits.

However, the ACA will not solve the healthcare cost problem. The cost problem is daunting. Ultimately that creates an insurmountable access problem – and threatens our entire economy.

The Centers for Medicare and Medicaid Services project national health expenditures at $2.8 trillion in 2012 — nearly

---

H.R. Brereton (Gubby) Barlow is President and Chief Executive Officer of Premera Blue Cross. The Premera family of companies provides health insurance and related services to 1.6 million people in Washington, Alaska, and Oregon. Barlow holds a Masters degree in business administration from the University of Cape Town and is a graduate of the Executive Management Program at the University of California at Los Angeles.

DEAR GOVERNOR:

18% of our national economy, averaging $8,937 for every man, woman and child, and far more of our economy than any other nation on earth.

Today, America's healthcare system is the fifth largest GDP on earth – as big as the economy of France. By 2020, after the ACA is fully implemented, officials estimate costs will rise to nearly $14,000 per capita – a 53 percent increase.

This trend is worrisome in its own right. Beyond threatening affordable access to healthcare, it now threatens the fate of our overall economy, as seen in financial scenarios published by the U.S. Congressional Budget Office.

In its scenario "which incorporates several changes to current law that are widely expected to occur or that would modify some provisions of law that might be difficult to sustain for a long period," the Congressional Budget Office assumes that the average level of past tax revenues (just under 20% of GDP) is likely to hold steady into the future.

However, federal spending, already outpacing revenues by about $1 trillion, is projected to rise over time as a share of GDP, creating a growing economic crisis fueled by spending above our means.

A closer look reveals that all other federal spending except healthcare and social security are *diminishing* as a share of the economy over time. However, federal healthcare spending is *ballooning*. After accounting for the growing interest payments on our federal debt driven by growing healthcare spending, total federal spending including interest approaches 34% of the U.S. economy by 2035 and accelerates from there.

Anatomy of a Crisis...

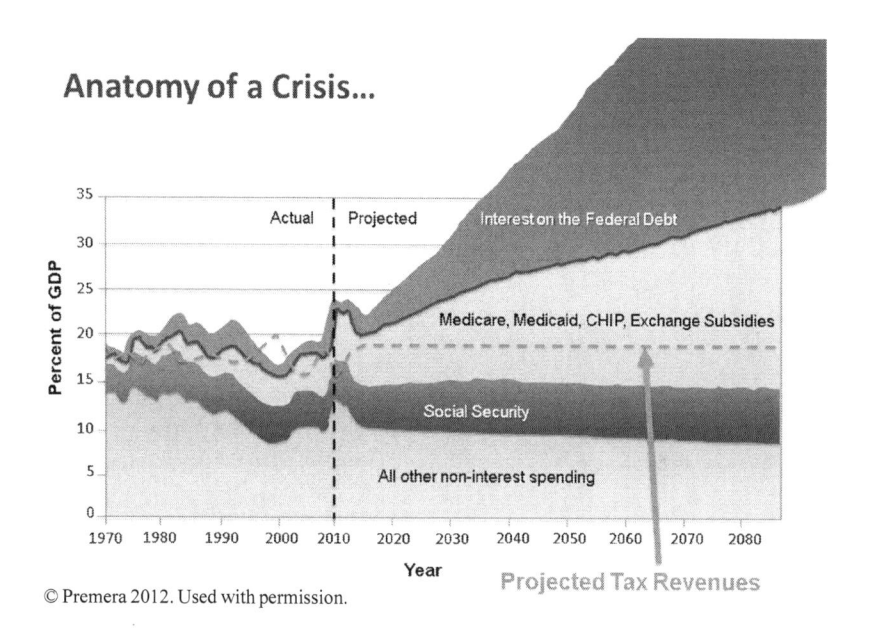

© Premera 2012. Used with permission.

Left unchecked, federal healthcare spending alone, coupled with interest on the debt, will bankrupt the country.

We know the underlying drivers: unhealthy lifestyles and an inefficient healthcare delivery system, aggravated by expensive new medical technologies. There is tremendous variation and waste in healthcare – even at the top academic medical centers.

One of the most telling anecdotes remains the Dartmouth study reviewing healthcare delivered to Medicare patients in the last six months of life. Researchers found that *depending on the medical center they used*, patients might spend about 11 days in the hospital – or nearly a month. They might see their doctor 20 times on average – or 82 times. Remember, by definition the outcome was identical: the patients expired. But the average amount of healthcare delivered certainly differed.

We know these variations in practice patterns can have a huge impact on cost. Let me offer three illustrations which sharpen the point.

In the Puget Sound area in 2011, the *average* cost for routine childbirth by one Puget Sound area medical group was about $9,000. Average cost charged by another was about $16,000. Both medical groups are prominent and well respected.

For annual diabetes treatment/management, average costs by medical group ranged from about $1,400 to about $3,000.

Average costs by medical group for back pain and degenerative joints ranged from about $2,200 to about $5,200. Again, these medical groups are all familiar and well respected—and the price ranges were typical, not the extremes.

In a well functioning market, consumers would ferret out those price differences and claim their reward. But healthcare is not a well functioning market.

Don't get me wrong: there are many activities to reward healthy lifestyles and more cost-effective care. Premera's Global Outcomes Contracting is just one example.

We're already collaborating with 1,500 Washington physicians to pay for healthcare differently – a shared savings approach that rewards them when their quality is up and their costs are lower than the market as a whole. We're also seeing results in our efforts to create a culture of health in our company and for our clients.

As to healthcare industry leadership, we are doing well in the Pacific Northwest. In fact, you may have seen the Spring 2012

PBS documentary on healthcare in America. The Northwest – and specifically work at The Everett Clinic, Group Health, Providence and Premera – has been cited as a national model. That's quite an honor.

Problem is, I don't *feel* like a national model.

Are we trying to make a difference? Of course. In truth, we fiddle around the edges. For all these efforts, healthcare costs continue to escalate.

The issue is that we are relying on the supply side of the healthcare market – doctors, hospitals government, insurers – to make accurate judgments about what customers really value. That is very hard to do anywhere, let alone with something as personal as healthcare.

Instead, we need to design a healthcare system that answers this simple question: what would patients actually buy if they were spending money out of their own health savings accounts?

We have to find a better way – a revolutionary way – to engage patients in the normal economic process of making trade-offs on where to spend their hard earned dollars.

Yes, we must shelter patients from financial devastation through insurance policies for major illness. But we must also give consumers real skin in the game. This has worked well for every other walk of economic life from cars to computers, even food, from the dawn of the supply and demand curve.

Many argue that it's wrong to think of healthcare as a competitive market; that healthcare is too complex, too precious, or that patients can't be expected to make trade-offs on matters of health and life.

That's condescending. Most importantly, it's untrue. For example, we see today, even in this opaque system, that when people buy their own high-deductible insurance and pick their own doctors, they make better economic decisions, which benefit themselves and society as a whole.

In studies of our own members, people with individual coverage who buy high-deductible insurance plans manage to use 15 percent less healthcare than the average of all of our customers. Meanwhile, employees of larger self-funded companies that offer richer benefits and lower deductibles use up to 18 percent more than average.

In other words, when people have little concern about their out of pocket expenses, they drive nearly 40 percent higher overall costs than those who do. Their more cost-conscious counterparts with individual coverage spend a lot less – and more importantly, have *similar health*, based on our analyses of relative health risk.

So, where do we go from here?

Health plans have an imperative to make it easier for consumers to see the true costs of care, and to make personal economic trade-offs. Once empowered, consumers will design the healthcare system they prefer. They will compel the healthcare finance and delivery system to transform itself – out of its own self interest.

Government has a crucial role: not in more top-down, command and control regulation, but by refocusing its efforts to facilitate a thriving marketplace – in the private sector *and* in Medicare, the single largest source of medical spending. As the nation's biggest insurer, Medicare dictates how our healthcare system operates.

Government's greatest opportunity for impact is to engage nearly 50 million Medicare beneficiaries, so they can be more deeply and meaningfully involved in making choices and making the trade-offs they do every day in other parts of life.

There are many proposals. One is from James Capretta, currently a Fellow with the Ethics & Public Policy Center. Mr. Capretta wants to supercharge the demand side, starting with Medicare.

He believes that if 50 million seniors can be transformed into savvy consumers, with a real stake in demanding more cost-effective healthcare, Medicare reform could be a huge watershed moment for Americans – a tipping point. His proposal involves premium supports – an approach that has bipartisan support.

If we are serious about creating a sustainable healthcare system, ultimately the ACA must change, too. It is unfortunate that rather than sensitizing and empowering consumers, the ACA has insulated people from the true costs of care further by lowering the deductibles and out of pocket maximums that insurers can set.

Billions of dollars are being directed to individuals through subsidies and other means: we need to redirect the dollars that are already going to be spent by *others* purportedly on consumers' behalf, and find ways to put the consumer in the driver's seat, creating a more direct opportunity for personal accountability and reward.

Yes, this is a difficult discussion, but the economic threat created by our trajectory of healthcare spending leaves us no realistic alternative.

In sum, we stand at a critical threshold with healthcare today. Our medical system borders on the miraculous. Beyond remarkable. But not sustainable. And our economy – and our children's future — now hang in the balance.

We don't need reform. We need a revolution. A revolutionary approach that fully engages the consumer and activates the demand side. And we need to show progress on this new course well within this decade.

Sincerely,

Gubby Barlow

ALASKA
IDAHO
OREGON
WASHINGTON

DAVID ROLF

President
SEIU Healthcare 775NW

Dear Governor,

Neither health care consumers, workers, nor our communities can afford to continue our fragmented, inefficient, uncoordinated approach to health care for low-income and vulnerable populations.

I have listened year after year as home care aides tell how their clients can't get the care they need in the medical system, how fragmented and uncoordinated care leads to poor health outcomes, and how adequate investment in a quality home and community based long-term care system would save billions of dollars in emergency room visits, hospitalizations, and skilled nursing facilities.

Home care aides provide personal care assistance such as

> *David Rolf is International Vice President of Service Employees International Union and President of SEIU Healthcare 775NW, and Chairs the SEIU Home Care Council. He also is Chair of the SEIU Healthcare NW Training Partnership, which provides basic and continuing career education to 43,000 home care aides each year in Washington State.*

medication management, transfer, bathing and meal preparation to seniors and people with disabilities to allow them to remain independent and live safely in their own homes and communities.

Home care is a strenuous and difficult job, and home care aides lift consumers and sometimes handle biomedical hazards, such as blood and human waste. These services are largely publicly funded through the Medicaid program and the workforce is comprised of disproportionately older and female workers.

Home care aides receive low wages, few (if any) benefits, and little job training or ongoing support. Nationally, home care aides earn an average of $9.49 per hour and nearly half of home care aides live in households earning below 200% of the federal poverty level income and receive one or more public benefits such as food stamps, Medicaid, housing, child care, and energy assistance.

While home care aides provide an invaluable service by keeping people at home and out of more costly institutions such as nursing homes and emergency rooms, they are rarely provided adequate training or support or treated as part of the medical team.

I frequently tell the story of being in Chicago a few years back and walking up a flight of stairs with a home care aide, who was about my age; a single, middle-aged mother earning just over the minimum wage and struggling with her own challenges with health, diet, and obesity. When we got to the top of the stairs she was extremely winded.

We entered her client's apartment and I sat in the kitchen with her, watching her prepare breakfast for her client. She made her bed-bound diabetic client a bowl of oatmeal with a stick of butter and a cup of sugar. Now, while I don't think she intended on killing her client, that bowl of oatmeal might have been enough to put even me into a diabetic coma.

This incident made me think about the difference that could be made if home care aides were treated as a real partner in the healthcare team, and trained and compensated accordingly. Integrating home care aides into the healthcare team could not only make poor meal preparation a thing of the past, but ultimately would improve health outcomes and quality of life for clients in a meaningful way.

Countless home care aides tell the story of the same shared experience about how they regularly are paid by Medicaid to drive their elderly or disabled clients to their doctors' appointments and then proceed to sit in the waiting room until the Medicare-funded appointment is complete.

Because coordinated care management for "dual eligibles" – often the sickest, most disabled, and most costly patients we treat – is the exception, not the rule, home care aides are rarely asked for input, even though it is this aide that frequently knows the consumer better than any other member of the healthcare team.

She may remember better than her client with dementia, or be less embarrassed than the patient to tell her doctor about increased incontinence episodes or falls or memory loss or prescription adherence. Yet rarely are home care aides involved in follow up and monitoring after the doctor visit.

Continuing this siloed approach that underutilizes the home care aide wastes resources and does nothing to enhance the quality of care and life for some of our most vulnerable citizens.

DEAR GOVERNOR:

Improving Care for the Poorest and Sickest Medicare Beneficiaries, the "Dual Eligibles"

The federal and state effort to transform care for the 9.2 million individuals in our country enrolled in both Medicaid and Medicare holds great potential, both in terms of human and financial stakes. Dually eligible individuals are many of our country's sickest and most vulnerable adults; their healthcare costs were about $319.5 billion in 2011.

Long-term supports and services account for sixty-nine percent of all Medicaid spending on the duals. Forty percent of the duals receive long-term care services, and about half of those receiving long-term care have a home care aide in the home on a regular basis.

These "dual eligibles" are all low income; many are elderly, but many others are young and often have physical or developmental disabilities. The heterogeneity and complexity of the "duals," highlights the need for approaches closely tied to the needs of the particular beneficiary. Although the dual eligibles constitute just 15 percent of Medicaid enrollees and 16 percent of Medicare enrollees, they account for 39 percent of all Medicaid spending and 27 percent of all Medicare spending.

All too often, the healthcare and other support services dually eligible individuals receive are fragmented and uncoordinated. Dual eligibles represent a formidable challenge, as both states and the federal government examine what can be done to improve the quality of the care they receive and better integrate the care paid for by both Medicare and Medicaid. Achieving these goals is also viewed as an opportunity for reaping cost savings for federal and state governments.

Home Care Aides Can Improve Care for Dual Eligibles

Home care aides generally spend 20-30 hours per week providing paid personal care support to a Medicaid client and are extremely well-positioned to play a role in improving care as part of a multidisciplinary healthcare team. These workers serve a small number of clients, have regular contact with dually eligible individuals in their own homes, develop trusting relationships with clients and their families, and are uniquely positioned to notice subtle changes in condition.

Given the significant percentage of dually eligible individuals with long-term services and supports needs, it is frequently the case that a home care aide knows the consumer better and has significantly more contact with them than any other member of the healthcare team. Yet in our current system, these workers are not treated as a valued part of the care team and are simply given a list of tasks to complete without being held responsible for improving health outcomes.

Home care aides have self-identified the positive role they could play as coordinators, advocates, and coaches to facilitate care and communication between the healthcare team, motivate and encourage consumers to follow a care plan, and act as an advocate for the consumer with other healthcare providers.

Successful approaches at care integration must include strategies for appropriately utilizing the direct care workers in the long-term care system and creating a team approach that crosses the silos between medical care, behavioral health, and long-term services and supports.

In order to make care coordination truly value-add for individuals with long-term services and supports needs, there must be a formal role for home care aides in the new healthcare models and a clear plan for enhanced direct care worker training and responsibilities with measurable health outcome metrics.

Now is a time for innovation! The Affordable Care Act and the increase in associated federal funding, has given us all – states, community organizations, healthcare advocates and providers – an unprecedented opportunity to think creatively and intentionally about the role that home care aides and other direct care workers can play as part of a care team in coordinating care and in improving health outcomes for dually eligible individuals.

Sincerely,

David Rolf

IDAHO

Scott Kreiling

President
Regence BlueShield of Idaho

Dear Governor,

We all have good reasons to be concerned about the cost of health care and insurance coverage. At Regence BlueShield of Idaho, we see first-hand how health care costs are rising because we pay our members' medical bills. For the sake of our members across the state who have pooled their funds to pay for care, and for other Idaho families and businesses, we all want to bring down costs.

From my seat as a nonprofit health insurer, the insurance marketplace over the last decade has painted a difficult picture. Health care's relentless cost inflation is holding America's health system hostage.

Health care costs have risen more than three times faster than

Scott is responsible for strategy and execution for the Regence BlueShield of Idaho consistent with the company's overall direction. He directs and guides statewide operations and market performance while representing and promoting Regence in business and civic arenas throughout the state. Scott serves on the Board of Directors for the Boise Metro Chamber of Commerce and chairs the Chamber's Healthcare Advisory Council.

wages, squeezing family budgets and imposing a burden on many employers.

Addressing costs

Contrary to popular belief, reducing health care spending is not a simple matter of lowering premium rates. That's like trying to limit what a gas station owner can charge when it's really the price of oil that drives what consumers pay at the pump. Premiums are driven by the very things we want insurance to cover: doctors, hospitals outpatient care and prescription drugs.

A key step toward making health care—and coverage—more affordable and accessible is understanding where the money goes—and why. A recent report from the newly founded Health Care Cost Institute (HCCI) takes a fresh look at the money trail. HCCI obtained and analyzed data from three billion health care claims provided by the nation's largest health plans. They examined three factors contributing to total spending: the volume of services consumed, the mix of services used, and the price per service.

The key finding? Prices are the driving factor for health care spending growth.

Consider:

- **Facility Trends.** The average facility price paid for a hospital stay was $14,662 in 2010, a 5.1 percent increase over 2009. The price for an emergency room visit climbed to $1,327 in 2010, an 11 percent hike.

- **Prescription Drugs.** Prescription drug prices grew 3 percent overall from an average of $80 per prescription in

2009 to $82 in 2010. However, brand name drug prices increased 13 percent from 2009 to 2010, while generic drug prices decreased by 6.3 percent.

- **Professional Services.** The overall price of professional procedures that include doctor visits, lab tests, and diagnostic imaging, increased 2.6 percent. Payments for office visits—to both primary care and specialist providers—grew by more than 5 percent.

We see similar trends reflected in our own claims data. While the recession has slowed the use of health care services, costs continued to rise, in some cases off-setting declining utilization.

Going forward, we're seeing utilization rates beginning to pick up again. Also, with major coverage expansions under The Affordable Care Act set to begin in 2014, the demand for medical services is expected to further accelerate.

Reducing costs through innovations in care

The cost component is clear. High health care costs are squeezing everyone: employers struggling to offer coverage and individuals trying to afford their own policies. We have to tackle costs, but at the same time, we can't forget about quality.

There are several policy areas to consider – population health, consumer engagement, payment reform, to name a few – but simply put, it's delivering the right care to the right people at the right time.

For example, in Washington state, Regence BlueShield, partnered with a major employer and medical providers to develop a pilot program aimed at improving employee health and productivity and reducing overall costs. Called the Intensive Outpatient Care Program (IOCP), it centered on the medical home concept and focused intensively on employees with multiple health issues.

Over two and a half years, we worked to test a way of paying for teams of doctors and nurses to intensively treat, coach and communicate with patients, which insurers conventionally have not done. Payment for care involved an unusual combination of both service and monthly fees.

The pilot program resulted in cost savings of 20 percent, primarily due to fewer hospitalizations and emergency room visits. By delivering highly-personalized, coordinated care, the program also achieved significant gains in employee health and productivity.

Today we've expanded the program across our markets, including Idaho. The IOCP model and others like it, shows that the private sector — including employers, insurers and medical professionals — is well-positioned to improve health care and reduce costs.

Access and choice affect affordability

As we've shown, getting a handle on health care costs isn't a one player game.

We need to work together to create positive change and that includes state and federal government. Like it or not, the Affordable Care Act has been upheld.

State health insurance exchanges – a key provision of the law – offer the potential to get more people protected by health care coverage which is essential to establishing an affordable, sustainable health care system for the long term.

Here in Idaho, a coalition of more than 45 small and large Idaho businesses, industry groups and chambers of commerce agrees. Lawmakers need to put aside their political differences and take a fresh look at setting up a market-driven exchange that would allow Idahoans the opportunity to shop and compare coverage.

Transparency and competitive choice have the power to not only transform how we shop for health care but begin shifting the very culture of health care in this country.

Transforming health care

It is every-day economics, in the daily lives of Idahoans and their employers, that dictates the need for an improved health care system, not politics. The power to transform health care is in our hands. The stakes are high and solving this crisis will demand the best in all of us.

Sincerely,

Scott Kreiling

DEAR GOVERNOR:

WASHINGTON

AARON KATZ

Principal Lecturer of Health Services and Global Health
University of Washington

Dear Governor,

The pioneers who drafted the Washington State Constitution were public health experts.

No, really. As far as we know, none of the 75 delegates to the Constitutional Convention of 1889 was an epidemiologist, but their words – "It is the paramount duty of the state to make ample provision for the education of all children" (Article IX) – show they understood that an educated public is fundamental to a healthy society. Today, we have a large body of research to support their wisdom.

How far we've strayed. In Washington State, since 2009 we've slashed nearly $5 billion from K-12 and higher education,

---

Aaron Katz teaches several health policy courses for graduate students in public health, health administration, and other UW programs, including in the Community Oriented Public Health Practice and Global Health MPH programs. He received the American Public Health Association's Award for Excellence in 2006 and the School of Public Health and Community Medicine's Outstanding Teaching Award in 2004.

jeopardizing the health and well-being of a generation of children and threatening to condemn a stellar system of public colleges and universities to a future of mediocrity.

This is shameful and avoidable. The next governor can do two things to reverse the harm and improve the health of all Washingtonians – make the case for additional tax revenues to support a quality educational system and redouble state efforts to reign in health care costs, which have the effect of crowding out education in the state budget.

The case for higher taxes is simple. U.S. Supreme Court Justice Oliver Wendell Holmes said it best: "Taxes are the price we pay for a civilized society." State government needs adequate income to provide a quality education system as well as meet other expectations we have as citizens, yet we've been increasingly starving it for the past 20 years through tax limiting initiatives and tax loopholes. We need a governor who will reverse this course.

Health care is more complicated.

State health care spending is increasing for two reasons. First, as employer-sponsored health insurance has eroded – the Great Recession has accelerated an existing long-term trend – Medicaid and other state-funding health insurance programs have filled the gap.

Second, the broader health care system is inherently inefficient and inflationary. So, for example, during the recession, even as the annual increase in overall national health care spending has dropped below 4%, the lowest in 50 years, prices of health care goods and services have risen much faster. What the state pays for health care is largely a product of those price increases; that is, state government is largely a "price taker."

Still, the State of Washington has been one of the most active states in seeking efficiencies in its regulation and purchase of health care services. It moved most acute care Medicaid beneficiaries into managed care plans in the 1990s, the vast majority of Basic Health clients are served by two highly managed plans, it has an aggressive Medicaid drug purchasing program and has been an innovator at trying to find efficient and effective ways of serving the most difficult patients, those with multiple, chronic diseases.

Certainly, more can be done along all these lines, but it's safe to say the potential to "save" money in state-purchased health care does not reach into the billions of dollars – a few hundreds of millions, perhaps, but not billions. And it is billions in savings that are necessary if Washington is to again become a leader in public education and if the economic burden of high health care costs on families and businesses is going to be eased.

The federal Affordable Care Act lays the groundwork for fixing the system, but it didn't go far enough; it did not include proven mechanisms to control health care spending. The experiences of many Western industrialized countries provide us with two basic models that will allow us to reign in health care spending.

First is what we might call the "public agency" model – like transportation or law enforcement, state government would pay for health care or health insurance for all its citizens with a budget set and controlled by the Legislature.

Funding would come from some combination of taxes and user fees (that is, premium shares, co-payments, etc.). This is the model used by Canada and the United Kingdom, among others.

The second approach is the "public utility" model. Here, rather than financing health care for everyone, the state sets up strong regulations of the health insurance industry so that it competes in ways that promote access, efficiency, and quality.

Think electricity or water, markets in which private enterprise can add value but not at expense of anyone's basic needs. Germany and the Netherlands have health care systems based on this "public utility" model.

We need a governor who will set aside economic theories that don't work in the real world of health care in favor of time-tested policies that do. These two evidence-based models provide the next governor with the opportunity to lead us toward real health care reform and, therefore, toward rebuilding our education system, the paramount duty of state government and the key to a healthy population.

Sincerely,

Aaron Katz

WASHINGTON

SCOTT ARMSTONG

President and Chief Executive Officer
Group Health Cooperative

Dear Governor,

There's no doubt that the Supreme Court's landmark ruling to uphold most of the provisions of the Affordable Care Act was a key milestone in the evolution of health reform in this country. But as important as the decision was, it was really just one single step in a process that started long before the Affordable Care Act passed and will continue for a long time to come.

What tended to get lost in all the speculation leading up the Court's decision, and the focus on the political implications afterward, was an important truth about how health care really works.

There's no doubt that federal policy plays a vital role in creating the framework for a health system that can provide affordable,

---

Scott Armstrong is President and CEO of Group Health Cooperative, one of the nation's largest consumer-governed health care systems. He has been with Group Health since 1986. Armstrong has nearly 30 years of experience in health care.

high-quality care to all Americans. That's why the decision to uphold the individual mandate mattered: it kept in place the federal structure for expanding health care coverage when the mandate goes into effect in 2014.

But what happens in Washington State is just as important as what goes on in Washington D.C.

For example, decisions that are made at the state level about how to implement provisions of the Affordable Care Act will go a long way toward determining whether citizens in this state who can't afford the care they need today get access to affordable, high-quality coverage in the future.

And ultimately, the decisions that affect our health the most are the ones we make every day when we consult with our doctor, or when we choose what to eat and how much to exercise. What really determines the quality and cost of medicine is the access people have to care, the procedures they choose, and how they manage their chronic conditions.

These are some of the challenges that local health care providers around the country are focused on today.

Washington State in particular has been a great laboratory for new ideas about how to make health care work better for local communities. For example, organizations such as Group Health, Virginia Mason, The Everett Clinic, and Providence Health Care of Spokane are leading efforts to build integrated systems that deliver better health and more affordable care. And the Puget Sound Health Alliance is providing information, so that people can make smart decisions about how they spend their health care dollars.

We don't have all the answers yet, but we've learned some important lessons. We know that lifelong health starts with a strong relationship between patients and primary care doctors. Treatment must take into account standards based on up-to-date medical research. Technology should connect patients and clinicians to each other and the information they need. And people must be actively involved in their own health, in the doctor's office and beyond.

We also know that how we pay for health care is hugely important. The traditional approach in this country—payment for each procedure—leads to a system that emphasizes treatment over prevention. Health care works best when doctors are paid to help people choose treatment that is best for them rather than the hospital or clinic's bottom line.

As we apply these lessons at Group Health, we've reduced emergency room visits by 29 percent and lowered the rate of some expensive elective procedures by 25 percent. Helping people manage their chronic conditions improves their quality of life and saves nearly $600 per patient each year.

These are great examples of how coordinated health care systems help people live healthier lives and control costs at the same time.

But for all the progress that Group Health and other organizations in the state are making toward care delivery improvements that lead to better care that costs less, the fact remains that health care coverage is still too expensive for far too many people in Washington State.

This is where the state policymakers can make a difference, particularly as they make decisions about key elements of the

DEAR GOVERNOR:

Washington Health Benefits Exchange.

The starting point for a successful Exchange is to make sure that as many people enroll as possible. This means it is critical that policymakers make it is easy for people to participate.

It's also important that people have access to transparent information about quality so they can make smart decisions about their care based on a clear understanding of value, and that there are provisions that ensure continuity of coverage as people move between Medicaid and the Exchange. The Puget Sound Health Alliance is a valuable model for how this can work.

There is another area where Washington State can influence the direction and pace of reform in local communities: through payment systems and health plan benefits within the care health programs that it controls.

Because Washington offers medical plans to state employees and pays for Medicaid coverage for eligible residents, it is one of the biggest purchasers of medical services in the state. By designing payments structures and health plan benefits to support efficient, high-value care, the state can nudge local health care providers toward innovations that have been proven to provide better outcomes at lower costs.

As policymakers begin to design the Washington Health Benefits Exchange, there are important opportunities to include similar requirements for health plans that choose to participate.

The truth is that it is going to take a long time and a lot of hard work to fix this country's broken health care system. As we move forward, the pressure to innovate and improve will increase and the rapid pace of change will continue.

The good news is that there is a lot we can do right here in Washington State to make a difference through local innovations that improve quality and lower costs.

Sincerely,

Scott Armstrong

DEAR GOVERNOR:

ALASKA
IDAHO
OREGON
WASHINGTON

DONALD FISHER

Chief Executive Officer
American Medical Group Association

Dear Governor,

Thank you for seeking input from our organization as you work to develop important health policy initiatives. While we appreciate the work that you are doing, we remain vitally concerned about our ability to continue to provide high-quality medical services in the current environment at both the federal and state levels.

The American Medical Group Association (AMGA) represents multi-specialty medical groups and other organized systems of care, including some of the nation's largest, most prestigious integrated health care delivery systems.

More specifically, AMGA represents 415 medical groups that employ nearly 125,000 physicians who annually treat more than 130 million patients in 49 states. A sizable number of these

---

Donald W. Fisher, Ph.D., is the President and Chief Executive Officer of the American Medical Group Association (AMGA). AMGA represents multi-specialty medical groups and other organized systems of care which deliver healthcare to 130 million patients in 49 states.

DEAR GOVERNOR:

patients are Medicare and Medicaid beneficiaries. We have a strong interest in providing high-quality medical services to these patients and developing a stable payment structure for physician services.

As you review value-based measures and practice arrangements that improve patient health outcomes and efficiency, we hope that you will find our comments concerning physician reimbursement under the federal health care programs, and care coordination to be helpful.

Physician Reimbursement Under Medicaid

As you well know, Medicaid is jointly funded by states and the federal government. Historically, reimbursement for physician services in Medicaid is significantly less than Medicare, let alone reimbursement from private payers. Alaska is a notable exception here.

AMGA has long taken the position that primary care is an important underpinning of our health care delivery system. Unfortunately, the shortage of primary care physicians is partially due to the current payment system.

Under fee-for-service payment mechanisms, primary care physicians are reimbursed for services based on the volume of care they deliver, rather than for care coordination, preventive care, and the use of protocols that promote high-quality patient-centered care.

I understand that you are wrestling with many financial decisions when it comes to the Medicaid program, particularly given the June 28, 2012, Supreme Court ruling. Although the Supreme Court of the United States upheld the provision expanding the number of people who qualify for Medicaid, a majority of the court said it would be unconstitutional to withhold existing Medicaid funds from states who do not comply.

By way of background, the Affordable Care Act, as signed into law by President Obama, allows states to expand Medicaid programs to cover individuals with incomes below 133 percent of the Federal Poverty Level. The law provides increased assistance to the states to help defray the costs of covering newly eligible beneficiaries.

However, this federal assistance is reduced in future years and does not apply to the 10-13 million individuals who were previously eligible for Medicaid but not enrolled. I expect that you will need to examine the income levels of your state residents, as well as the state budget from both a near-term and long-term perspective when making this important decision.

We recognize that the state is experiencing significant fiscal challenges, and that you may need to consider opting out of the Medicaid expansion – as the state will ultimately be required to finance part of it. If you decide to opt-out of the Medicaid expansion, certain low-income residents could be significantly impacted.

As you know, state health insurance exchange subsidies are available to individuals between 100 percent and 400 percent of the Federal Poverty Level. However, individuals with incomes below 100 percent of the Federal Poverty Level are ineligible for the subsidies -- as the law assumed that these residents would enroll in Medicaid. It is possible that these residents will have little or no health insurance options – as they will be ineligible for subsidies as well as Medicaid.

DEAR GOVERNOR:

The Act also included a provision that will raise Medicaid payment rates for certain primary care services to what Medicare pays for the same services in 2013 and 2014. This temporary payment increase, funded entirely with federal dollars, will certainly strengthen access to primary care services for existing and newly eligible Medicaid beneficiaries, but what will happen in 2015?

We recognize that the state faces a significant decision when it comes to Medicaid expansion. We also understand that the state is experiencing serious budgetary challenges and will continue to face significant fiscal issues when it comes to Medicaid.

Many states have enacted efforts to help control Medicaid spending; however, it is my hope that this short-term reimbursement increase will serve as a catalyst to achieving broader Medicaid reform.

I hope that you will take advantage of this two-year time period and explore various alternative Medicaid payment models.

You may want to consider recalibrating Medicaid payments to reward providers for certain activities, such as quality measurement and improvement activities; care coordination; and use of information technology and evidence-based medicine.

You may also want to consider advanced primary care models, such as Accountable Care Organizations (ACOs).

I believe that the increased Medicaid reimbursement in 2013 and 2014 provides you with an incredible opportunity to consider ways to completely transform the Medicaid program. AMGA members stand ready to serve as a resource as you examine Medicaid reimbursement solutions.

Care Coordination

AMGA members put a strong emphasis on coordinating the care of their patients, a service that is generally not reimbursable under existing payment methodologies, yet has shown great potential to reduce expenditures while improving patient care.

We applaud federal initiatives, such as ACOs, and private sector initiatives that provide opportunities for the most efficient and high-quality provider organizations to share in the savings they generate. But more needs to be done.

A 2009 Annals of Internal Medicine article examined the fee-for service Medicare program and found that the typical primary care doctor may need to coordinate care with 229 doctors across 117 different practices.[1]

The same article found that Medicare beneficiaries typically see seven different physicians from four different practices in a given year, and the care of patients with multiple chronic illnesses is even more fragmented.

High-performing health systems, multi-specialty medical groups, and other organized systems of care are the most effective and efficient delivery system model to coordinate care and provide high-quality, patient-centered health care to Americans. As such, state and national policies should work to stimulate formation, foster growth, and support development of organized systems of care.

---

[1] Honagmai H. Pham, MD, MPH; Ann S. O'Malley, MD, MPH; Peter B. Bach, MD, MAPP; Cynthia Saiontz-Martinez, ScM; and Deborah Schrag, MD, MPH. (2009). "Primary Care Physicians' Links to Other Physicians Through Medicare Patients: The Scope of Care Coordination." Annals of Internal Medicine (2009).

DEAR GOVERNOR:

AMGA members understand that patients often see multiple providers across different care settings. We believe that it is critical for providers to share clinical information with other providers, monitor patient status between visits, and fully communicate about self-care. Without such care management, patients are likely to be frustrated, medical errors are more likely to occur, and unnecessary utilization of medical services will take place.

That is why AMGA members are committed to coordinating care across patient conditions, services, and settings over time.

Many AMGA members have been early adopters of health information technology, which assists in the implementation of quality measurement and improvement activities. This important technology helps AMGA members improve health care quality and reduce costs.

It also allows AMGA members the ability to gather ongoing patient data, develop care plans, and analyze health care information that can be translated into actionable, coordinated, evidence-based practice.

Moreover, health information technology allows AMGA members to engage in data comparison efforts, which help multi-specialty medical groups, and other organized systems of care, discover new clinical processes and cost saving mechanisms.

Studies suggest that multi-specialty groups and other organized systems of care are more likely to use care management processes and may use fewer resources. Medical groups are more likely to invest in health information technology, form teams of providers, collect and analyze data, and provide direct physician feedback on clinical care.

Further, evidence shows there is greater collaboration among physician specialties and allied health professionals in large multi-specialty medical groups, which is a key component to successful care coordination. This collaboration leads to improved quality and reduced costs.

An article published in Health Affairs demonstrated that patients cared for in a multi-specialty medical group or other organized systems of care received higher quality care at a lower cost.[2]

The study collected ambulatory claims in 22 Hospital Referral Regions comparing data from physicians practicing in multi-specialty medical groups, and physicians not affiliated with multi-specialty medical groups.

The authors found within the same referral area, Medicare beneficiaries cared for by physicians practicing in multi-specialty medical groups received 5-15 percent higher quality of care at a cost that was $272 (3.6 percent) lower.

Quite simply, it is easier to coordinate the care of patients who receive care in multi- specialty medical groups and other organized systems of care.

These findings provide strong support for the multi-specialty medical group and other organized system of care model that puts a strong emphasis on care coordination.

---

[2] William B Weeks, Daniel J. Gottlieb, David E. Nyweidi, Jason M. Sutherland, Julie Bynum, Lawrence P. Casalino, Robin R. Gillies, Stephen M. Shortell, and Elliot S. Fisher. "Higher Health Care Quality and Bigger Savings Found At Large Multispecialty Medical Groups." Health Affairs, 29:5, 991-997. (May 2010).

The authors estimate that the 3.6 percent cost savings across all physicians could save Medicare $15 billion in a year or $150 billion over a decade, a sizeable contribution to the almost $1 trillion Affordable Care Act.

Summary and Conclusion

In summary, AMGA recommends that you work to:

- Explore innovative payment models in the Medicaid program, especially in 2013-2014 that will reward integration,

- And incentivize care coordination through innovative payment models that reward this desirable activity.

Thank you for taking time to consider some of our views. I stand ready to work with you and members of the state legislature on health care policy issues.

Sincerely,

Donald W. Fisher, Ph.D., CAE

ALASKA
IDAHO
OREGON
WASHINGTON

TOM FRITZ

Chief Executive Officer
Inland Northwest Health Services

Dear Governor,

Following the Supreme Court's landmark ruling to uphold the Patient Protection and Affordable Care Act, many reform decisions come down to states implementing the law. While the impact of that ruling is still to be recognized over the months and years ahead, Washington is in a position to ensure healthcare decisions implemented throughout our state are positioned to improve care while creating efficiencies in the delivery of care and ultimately lowering costs throughout the system. Many of those initiatives will be greatly supported by health information technology solutions which have been proven to increase efficiency and lower costs.

Encourage Electronic Health Information Technology Collaborations

It is estimated that our nation is spending $2.7 trillion annually on

Tom Fritz is Chief Executive Officer of Inland Northwest Services based in Spokane, Washington. The organization is regarded as one of the leading health information exchange services in the nation, connecting hospital systems and community providers across three states.

DEAR GOVERNOR:

healthcare, making the benefits of electronic health information technology even more compelling: reduced medical errors, decreased redundancy in tests, improved workflows, faster claims processing, decreased lengths of stay and improved clinical decision-making – all of which ultimately reduce costs in healthcare.

Medical communities throughout the Spokane Hospital Referral Region have worked hard to further the adoption of electronic data utilization. At more than 65% adoption, our region is nationally recognized for using technology to improve patient safety and clinical outcomes.

Twelve hospitals utilizing certified technology solutions from Inland Northwest Health Services (INHS) were among the first in Washington to successfully attest and receive more than $40 million through the Medicare Electronic Health Record (EHR) Incentive Program for meeting Meaningful Use Stage 1 criteria.

Yet the total hospital numbers achieving attestation nationwide remain low. Washington has opportunities to maximize federal dollars at the state level for further technology adoption.

Our region has also benefited in working collaboratively with state and national organizations to further health technology solutions that improve care and reduce costs:

- INHS is working with the Social Security Administration to shorten disability claims decisions by extracting pertinent data from clinical electronic medical record systems and sending data electronically to SSA through the Nationwide Health Information Network.

- In collaboration with the Spokane Veterans Affairs Medical Center and Fairchild Air Force Base, INHS is participating in the national Virtual Lifetime Electronic Record (VLER) pilot to create a consolidated, coherent, consistent view of electronic health records for Active Duty Services Members and Veterans, regardless of where they receive care.

- To support tracking of population health, INHS is working with the Centers for Disease Control and Prevention, Washington and Idaho state departments of health and the Spokane Regional Health District.

- Our region was selected as one of 17 Beacon Communities in the nation to lead a collaborative regional effort to address reducing costs and improving health outcomes for patients with Type 2 diabetes through shared technology and care coordination best practices.

- A state program of the Washington Department of Labor & Industries the Centers of Occupational Health & Education (COHE) utilizes occupational health best practices when treating injured workers as well as technology tools that improve communication between providers, employers and injured workers. COHE health care providers have 35% less time loss cases at 90 days post-injury, 30% less at 12 months, and 46% less at 24 months – compared to non-COHE providers.

    » The percentage of time loss disability claims over 90 days is 4.7% for Eastern Washington COHE (statewide average is 5.8%); and 6.7% for claims over 30 days time loss (statewide average is 10.4%)

    » Nearly $15 million annually is saved in eastern Washington communities, from direct medical and disability costs

As governor, we ask that you continue to encourage public-private collaborations for the benefit of our citizens.

Ensure Clinical Information is Shared

Spokane resident, Lisa, recently shared her frustrations with our health care system. "As a mom of three and a caregiver for my husband and our parents, I'm the one who is coordinating the communication and care between the different doctors my family sees because their electronic systems don't talk to one another. Shouldn't that be their job?"

Lisa's story is all too common and shows that technology has a long way to go to connect disparate health systems. A study conducted in June, 2012 by Robinson Research, and commissioned by INHS, showed that of 400 respondents in the Spokane region, the average number of doctors or care providers seen in the past year by the same patient was over three. This underscores the need for coordination and communication between providers who may not be in the same integrated delivery network.

While integrated models of care can greatly benefit patients, they only work if patients stay within that health delivery network. If Lisa or a family member, for example, goes outside their health delivery system, important health information may not be able to be electronically shared and care may be impacted.

To ensure patients don't lose the value that comes from providers sharing critical health information, we encourage you to implement policies that are consistent with federal initiatives, making healthcare technology systems interoperable and supporting more than health data exchange. For the benefit of patients and caregivers like Lisa and her family, we can't afford not to share critical health information.

Inform and Engage Consumers

Sixty-one year old Doreen is reassured by her provider's ability to access test results and review trends in her care over the last several visits, however she is frustrated that she can't do so herself.

"I like my provider, but because of how many patients he sees in a day, he only has a few minutes to explain things to me. I would enjoy being able to review my health record before or after the visit and from the comfort of my home."

Meaningful Use funds will help drive healthcare organizations to provide patients e-communication and access to important health information. However, the fundamental question is who ultimately owns patients' health data.

We should all agree that health information and data is owned by the patient.

As governor, I ask that your administration take the lead on educating patients on the ownership of their electronic health data and the benefits of electronic health records. Patients like Doreen will be more informed and have access to their health information.

Additionally, it is essential that patients are educated consumers regarding their healthcare. We can all agree that healthcare is in need of reform. Innovative technologies and sharing of data through health information exchanges are part of the equation.

Additionally, we must educate our state's citizens about the true costs of healthcare, their role in managing those costs and the benefits to them as a patient and the system as a whole.

DEAR GOVERNOR:

Collaboration Drives Innovative Healthcare

INHS, founded on a mission of collaboration to reduce costs and improve health outcomes, remains focused on how to best serve patients and our community, ensuring continuation of the benefits that have been created over the last 15 years through the advancements of health information technology solutions.

Our entire healthcare community must continue to work together, along with patients, purchasers, regional and national organizations, to further health information technology solutions for the benefits of the people we serve.

INHS looks forward to working with you and your administration to encourage collaborations and create additional opportunities for improved, coordinated and quality care.

In commitment to Washington's health,

Tom Fritz

IDAHO

TIMOTHY BROWN

Executive Director
Terry Reilly

Dear Governor,

It is time for Idaho's leadership to start working toward effective solutions to our broken healthcare system.

For the past 10 years, the staff and volunteers at Terry Reilly have resorted to organizing a bike tour, the Bob LeBow Bike Tour, to raise money to help cover the cost of providing quality healthcare to Idaho's population lacking health insurance and the resources to pay for their care. Is this really how healthcare should operate in Idaho? I believe we can do better.

While the Affordable Care Act is not necessarily how you or I would have approached remaking our healthcare system, it is the framework in which we must now operate. I believe it is now time for you to bring together Idaho's legislature and healthcare

Tim Brown has served as the Executive Director of Terry Reilly since early 2009. He has extensive experience in community health and non-profit management. Tim earned a B.A. in Anthropology from Franklin Pierce University and M.A. in Sociology and Anthropology from the American University in Cairo. When he is not working, Tim and his wife Dalia enjoy traveling both near and far.

DEAR GOVERNOR:

leaders to find ways for Idaho to make the Affordable Care Act work for Idaho.

There are opportunities within this legislation that can help drive improvement in both the delivery of care and the long-term health outcomes of Idahoans.

The two major opportunities before us that require your leadership are:

- The expansion of Medicaid – more than 100,000 Idahoans have the opportunity to qualify under the planned Medicaid expansion. Yes, the Supreme Court has ruled that threatening to cut existing funding for not adopting the expansion is not allowable, but not embracing the proposed expansion would hurt Idahoans. Under the Affordable Care Act, the federal government will cover 100 percent of the expansion through 2016. Idahoans are already paying for a lot of this care through the County and State Indigent Care Funds – expanding Medicaid will provide individuals the opportunity to access care proactively rather than waiting until they have experienced a health crisis and accumulated significant healthcare related debts. Our shared goal should be to drive down healthcare costs; expanding coverage should allow individuals to access care while initially the costs of the care will be covered through the Affordable Care Act.

- The Health Insurance Exchange – the creation of an Idaho Health Insurance Exchange has the potential to help control costs, improve access to health insurance, especially for individuals who are self-employed, while improving transparency and accountability. Idaho needs to adopt an exchange. The exchange will facilitate more competition within the insurance marketplace and provide individuals with more options. An Idaho exchange will force insurers to compete for their consumers based on value. Yes, operating the exchange will cost money, but if designed correctly, by Idaho, for Idaho, we should be able to keep costs manageable and ensure the exchange is responsive to local shifting needs.

There are also challenges that the Affordable Care Act creates for Idaho, that need your leadership to develop effective solutions.

These challenges include:

- We are going to need more healthcare providers. We need to continue and expand our investment in health professional training programs. We need these programs to grow their focus on training professionals for careers in rural parts of Idaho. We also need to develop a robust State loan repayment program – most other states already have such programs in place while Idaho has failed to compete.

- We need effective plans to control our healthcare costs. We need to invest in prevention and early intervention. We need to dismantle our County and State Indigent funds and invest in providing education; early intervention and work towards ensuring we are providing care at the appropriate, most cost effective level possible. We need to place the incentives in the correct places within the system, so we encourage patients and providers to access and deliver care at the most cost effective level of care possible.

These challenges need to be addressed immediately. Investing in these changes is not an endorsement of the Affordable Care Act; they are an investment in Idahoans. Idaho cannot and will not be able to attract the business and individuals needed to grow our economy and society, if we don't have a healthy population. The days of organizing bike tours to pay for our healthcare delivery needs to come to an end.

We have the opportunity to create an effective healthcare delivery system for the people of Idaho. Let's not miss this opportunity.

Sincerely,

Tim Brown

OREGON

MAGGIE BENNINGTON-DAVIS

Chief Medical and Operating Officer
Cascadia Behavioral Healthcare

Dear Governor,

I am excited about health transformation in Oregon. You have done a tremendous job emphasizing that both health care delivery, and health care financing, need a complete overhaul. I would add what we deliver in health care also needs changing.

Poverty, childhood trauma, loneliness, unaddressed depression and anxiety, substance use – these are major drivers of poor-health. Community behavioral health understands this.

Comprehensive community mental health programs, described by President Kennedy in the 1960's, took a systems approach to ensuring mental health treatment for people with serious mental illness. Although these programs never realized their potential because they were never adequately funded, health strategists can learn from the concepts. If the architects of our health

> *Dr. Maggie Bennington-Davis is currently Chief Medical and Operating Officer for Cascadia BHC in Portland, Oregon, which serves more than 12,000 children, teens, adults, and seniors annually in a broad continuum of services. Prior to Cascadia, Maggie served as Psychiatry Medical Director for a regional medical center (Salem Hospital), as well as hospital Chief of Staff.*

system aren't aware of these programs, there is a high risk of losing what little of this precious resource remains. I often observe that the hospital-based, physician-centric view of healthcare doesn't know what it doesn't know.

Comprehensive community-based behavioral health care includes crisis, sub acute, residential, housing, outreach, and clinic-based mental health and addiction services across the age spectrum. There is fragmentation and isolation of funding and policy for many services in behavioral health: residential services and crisis services in the Tri-County area are not integrated into the Coordinated Care Organizations (CCO); policy and oversight for residential, housing, and crisis services are at County and State levels; jail mental health care has not been integrated into the Tri-County plan. The "system" therefore will remain fragmented and wasteful – both in terms of health and costs.

There is a strong link between social supports like housing, jail alternatives, assistance obtaining benefits and mental health (we are learning that we do not need the modifier of "mental" – these things have a strong correlation with health in general). In order to improve health and decrease costs, we must create supports for people to adopt healthy behaviors, which have little to do with the typical physician visit. Our new CCOs are still very much focused on meetings between people and their physician, rather than on what improves health behaviors.

Community-based behavioral healthcare understands that engaging people, not just in services, but in healthy behaviors is the key to improving health. People with lived experienced (referred to as "peers") are the best people to engage others in understanding their own health, tapping their own strengths, changing bad habits, and maneuvering the system(s) that can best support them. Community-based behavioral healthcare has long understood the need for an "alternative" workforce, and has learned to efficiently and cost-effectively use its medical staff – psychiatrists, nurse practitioners, and nurses – but the mainstays of its services are case managers, therapists, and peers.

Oregon's plan calls for integration of behavioral health and primary healthcare – again, an essential element, but one not completely fleshed out. Currently, most health planners assume that "integration" means having a mental health professional embedded in primary care. For thousands of people with serious mental illness, this is not enough. For those thousands of people with serious mental illness, a health home is better situated outside the walls of primary care.

Meeting people where they are – on park benches, in shelters, under bridges – has long been a specialty of community based behavioral health. In order to improve health, we must create integration of primary care into already-existing community behavioral healthcare, as well as the reverse.

State and federal policies have failed to expedite these concepts – and in some cases are barriers. Oregon's "Medical Home" Act describes and requires primary medical care as the main instrument of health, and practically discourages community mental health centers from becoming health homes.

This is short-sighted. At the federal level, "meaningful use" fails to incentivize community behavioral health by focusing entirely on physician use of electronic health records. Yet, community behavioral health has been financially starved for decades, and information technology is expensive. It is costly both in terms of systems redesign and health to delay providing infrastructure to incorporate community behavioral health resources into the efforts of coordination and creation of health homes. It is unrealistic to think existing community behavioral health centers can transform without resources, and wasteful not to transform.

Ironically, in the midst of the promising reforms that Oregon has undertaken, community behavioral health budgets in Portland are once again being cut dramatically. These already-underfunded, inexpensive, effective services are not only the safety net for Oregon's most vulnerable citizens, they reduce the need for high-cost services such as hospitalization, and reduce unwanted and unnecessary interactions with police (that inevitably result in ER visits or jail).

The latest cut is seven million dollars from the Portland area, and will likely cause needed programs to shrink or close – ultimately costing the "system" more in high-level service costs and in the need to re-build these programs when the new system realizes their necessity.

In summary, given that health does not occur in the doctor's office, and unrecognized/unaddressed mental illness and substance abuse are major cost and illness drivers, I'd like you to consider:

- Integration is not just placing a mental health professional in primary care – it is much more radical than that, and you must ensure that State (and as much as you can, federal) policies facilitate integration (or - at the least - not block it).

- Community-based behavioral healthcare addresses health behaviors, uses an "alternative" workforce that is multi-disciplinary, and creates a person's health home where the person is; strategists for the new healthcare system should borrow the concepts.

- Community-based behavioral healthcare is (chronically)

underfunded, not able/incentivized to create develop the information technology for care coordination, and not able/incentivized/supported to integrate primary care into services.

- Community-based behavioral healthcare includes a comprehensive and coordinated spectrum of services but has been fragmented with isolated and complex funding streams, policies, and oversight; the new CCOs are at risk of perpetuating and even worsening that situation.

- Current over-spending on Medicaid high-end specialty medical services are causing cuts in lower-cost, primary care services which will increase the use of costly hospital services and cause safety-net programs to close.

So, Governor, carry on! I am proud to be a physician in Oregon during this time of unprecedented change, and glad you are at the helm.

Sincerely,

Maggie Bennington-Davis, M.D.

DEAR GOVERNOR:

IDAHO

JOHN L. HOOPES

Chief Executive Officer
Caribou Memorial Hospital

Dear Governor,

I have been the CEO of small rural hospitals with attached nursing homes and primary care clinics since 1979, in Oregon, Arizona and Idaho.

For the past decade, our organization in Soda Springs, Idaho, has been a critical access hospital, our clinic is a rural health clinic, and we have done very well.

Because of our county's less than 7,000 population, and with only five employed local providers, who staff our ER, hospital and clinics on a 24/7 basis, we know almost everyone for whom we have the privilege of providing cradle-to-the-grave healthcare.

John L. Hoopes is CEO at Caribou Memorial Hospital, Soda Springs, Idaho. He brings 12 years of hospital administration experience to his current position at Caribou, but he's been working with county hospitals for 30 years. John has a Masters degree in hospital administration.

DEAR GOVERNOR:

I am writing this after reading the June 11, 2012 cover story, "How to Die" in Time magazine, by Joe Klein. It was a well-written, first-hand account of the passing of his parents. We have 30 nursing home beds attached to our hospital and this process unfolds several times a month, for people we have cared for and known for years.

Compared with our healthcare organization, Geisinger, the system in Pennsylvania with 2.6 million patients that Klein describes, is huge. However, their modus operandi is not unique. What Klein describes sounds a lot like small-town—where everyone knows everyone—medicine and institutional care.

Just as Soda Springs isn't big enough to support a Wal-Mart or McDonalds, we also can't support the overhead that Geisinger employs, but our healthcare is excellent, efficient, compassionate, and our charges are well below the national average. Our doctors and nurses, who know our patients like family, function like the "case managers" Klein describes.

Klein writes that salaried doctors are not motivated to do more for patients than patients really need, because these doctors aren't paid based on the services they perform.

Our salaried doctors only receive bonuses when the "bottom lines" of their clinics are positive. If they keep the cost of doing business down and see more patients, they could get bonuses.

We are county-owned, but get no funding from local taxes, and have managed to re-invest in our infrastructure. Last year we dedicated a $2.5 million new surgery addition we paid for with cash. Our organization is debt free and profitable.

We are too small to be an Accountable Care Organization, as

Klein describes, and no one is trying to form one in Southeastern Idaho. Even though this isn't about ACOs, big hospitals in Idaho are trying to get legislation to designate trauma centers, so they can be paid more. We want small hospitals to be able to continue to provide emergency care for our patients before we transfer them.

I hope that, if these ACOs don't survive, we can continue to provide care for our local residents in the ways we have been successful, and not be forced into being part of a system, dictated by big hospitals or insurers, and certainly not government bureaucracies.

Klein credits the computerization of medical records for Geisinger's success. Unfortunately, we have not yet had success with our electronic health record; it has only been an expensive burden, so far. Our physicians were already efficient in documenting what they do, so using the EHR has slowed them down a lot.

We spent two years trying to decide which EHR to buy, and only chose one because we have been using their financial software for 15 years.

We learned after our new EHR was installed that the platform on which it operates doesn't interface well with our lab equipment and financial program, and that nursing has to create their own assessments.

Along with all this, we will soon have to replace the financial system to interface with the new EHR. This may cost more than if we would have just started over with a new system, although we don't know of a better one. The government's touted incentives may only reimburse us about 51% of the cost of our EHR, and nothing for the headaches it's causing.

DEAR GOVERNOR:

We have reported quality indicators, using national criteria, for years on a monthly dashboard. However, since implementing the EHR, for which we have met "meaningful use," we can't even extract the data for the indicators. Other small-rural hospitals in our local 13-hospital cooperative have had the same experiences we have, and are just as frustrated.

Our organization provides excellent, well-coordinated care, and our population is very healthy, compared with national norms. Charges for our services are low, compared with national norms.

The biggest problem is that it is not equitable for our well insured majority, thanks to our local industries and businesses, to subsidize the minority, who isn't insured, either because they can't or won't pay for it. Some people won't even apply for Medicaid or county indigence, because they don't want liens placed on their assets.

Several times a month I am handed a pile of accounts and asked to sign over those who promised, but have not made payments, to collection agencies. This is painful for me, because I know most of these people.

I don't feel so badly for those who have new pickups, 4 wheelers and snowmobiles, and make payments to keep their "toys," but don't make their doctor and/or hospital payments. However, I know good, honest people who don't make enough to buy health insurance and can't qualify for assistance.

Regardless of what happens after the election, there must be changes in the way healthcare is financed. We obviously can't continue to support the inequitable financing system we now have.

We just hope that in our small-rural area we can keep all of the great things we enjoy that are working so well, and not be forced into a mandated, bureaucratic system that makes things worse, or more expensive, for the majority of our residents.

Sincerely,

John L. Hoopes

DEAR GOVERNOR:

OREGON

MELINDA MULLER

Clinical Vice President, Primary Care
Legacy Medical Group
Legacy Health

Dear Governor,

Successful health reform is going to rely on the effective use of one of the scarcest resources in the health system: primary care providers. Much has been written about the importance of primary care and its role in improving quality and reducing costs in the system. However, to realize the potential of effective primary care, investments need to be made first.

Primary care providers are stuck on the treadmill of running from patient to patient to make a living. My experience the last 5 years in transforming our primary care services has shown me that if you want real transformation, you need to spend money to save money.

Melinda Muller, MD is recognized by the National Committee for Quality Assurance (NCQA) and the American Diabetes Association (ADA) for providing quality care to her patients with diabetes.

Small investments give the primary care providers and clinics the time to look at their workflow processes and evaluate how they could perform that work differently. That can free up time for the work that is going to make a real difference: proactive outreach to patients for their preventative health needs and management of chronic diseases.

Providing a small ($5-10k) stipend allows a provider to block out a few patient appointments so providers and staff can meet regularly to plan and evaluate new workflows. This will make a large difference in the success of those changes. That protected time is important. If you expect people to do this on top of their regular workload, it is doomed to failure.

The other place investment is key is payment for services and incenting the right work. Primary care is between a rock and a hard place: providers need to see patients to stay in business in the current payment structure. If you change the work to decrease office visits (i.e. using email or phone visits or communication) you get more proactive, patient centered care, but this works against the provider in the current system.

At the same time, payers are saying if you change your work and give us better outcomes we will pay you differently, but aren't recognizing that most clinics can't find the time or resources to allow the changes to be made. It's a Catch 22 for primary care providers in this transition period.

Recognition of the startup costs and funding those needs are essential for success. The clinics that have been successful in navigating this transition period are those that have received some seed money to allow the providers to take some risks, to make some changes while staying in business. After all, each independent clinic is a small business with all the requirements that go along with running a business.

Another large issue for primary care providers that impacts their work and well-being is access to behavioral health providers. Primary care providers deliver 75% of depression care in the United States.

It makes sense for primary care providers to deliver that care within the context of caring for the whole patient.

However, patients often require resources that are outside the scope and training of the primary care provider. In addition, as noted above, it's hard to do appropriate behavioral and mental health care within a 15 minute office visit. Taking longer for a visit reduces volume, and therefore potentially income.

Successful models of behavioral health integration can be found throughout the country for patients with complex mental health disorders. These include co-location of behavioral health within primary care or co-location of primary care within behavioral health. It doesn't take great resources to make a large impact on patients.

It has been demonstrated that adding a social worker to a primary care clinic can impact unnecessary emergency room visits significantly – a reduction of 20% in some cases. This has positive downstream effects on costs, quality and satisfaction. The limiting factor, again, is the current payment system which carves out mental health into separate networks.

For true transformation, experimentation and innovation needs to go beyond the care delivery model. Much is happening in that arena, and the work is picking up speed. What is slowing the work down is the often glacial rate of payment reform changes.

DEAR GOVERNOR:

I recognize that whenever we talk about money things get complicated, and I also recognize that there isn't a blank check. People need to be held accountable for their processes and outcomes, so as not to waste money.

However, I believe transformation can be accelerated significantly by small focused investments of money. I have seen it work within my own clinic and I know that the primary care community is hungry for the change.

Sincerely,

Melinda Muller

ALASKA

Marilyn Kasmar

Former Chief Executive Officer
Alaska Primary Care Association

Dear Governor,

A lifelong Alaskan, I've worked as a registered nurse on the front lines of health care since 1982.

I've worked in flight nursing, neonatal intensive care, labor and delivery, and high-risk prenatal. I've also worked as an administrator, and for the last 16 years as the CEO of a member and policy organization that serves and supports Alaska's community health centers.

Through the years, I've worked with people in rural and urban, hospital and clinic, and tribal and non-tribal settings, and with people from all walks of life. I'm also the mother of two kids.

It's with my kids in mind that I write to you today. I've become

Marilyn Kasmar served as the CEO of the Alaska Primary Care Association (APCA) from 1996 - 2012. APCA is a not-for-profit organization founded in 1995 working to promote, expand and optimize primary care access so that all Alaskans will have that access, including the underserved. She is involved in numerous professional boards, coalitions and workgroups at the national, regional, state and local levels.

deeply concerned about the future of health care for them, and whether or not they are going to be able to access and afford it when they need it in the coming years. A lot of other people I talk with are experiencing the same trepidation for their children and grandchildren.

On behalf of my kids, I'd like to share with you what I see as some of the concerns facing health care today, and what we need to focus on going forward to realign for success.

We all need health care at some point in our lives. We need it in acute times, when we've suffered an accident, a bug, or have been beset by something unfortunate like cancer, but we also need it on a preventive basis, as it helps us live better and serve society more effectively as strong, productive human beings. When we need it, we need it to be of good quality, and affordable.

Due to a multitude of complex factors, the health care system as a whole has evolved to the point where it's unsustainable, and to where the ability to access it is becoming unaffordable for employers and individuals alike. Uncorrected, this will erode us as a society.

Regardless of how people feel about whether or not health care is a right or a privilege, the fact is that as a people, we are as strong as our weakest link.

From a practical and philosophical standpoint, health care needs to be available and affordable to protect the health of us all. A strong and healthy people are the foundation of a powerful, robust and thriving society. If that foundation breaks down, over time it will negatively affect each of us.

Not one to think government should take a role where private enterprise should be, I've come to believe that when it comes to health care, the people need government to step up. Private enterprise is not serving the people well, and the people are deteriorating and dying as a result.

How do we realign to get back on the right track?

In the past, I have worked with others to develop a set of guiding principles for this conversation. I share them here.

- **Accessibility:** Alaska needs to establish and maintain a primary care system (medical, dental, vision and behavioral health) that is accessible to everyone, including those who need it but can't pay for it at the time they need it.

- **Primary Care as the Basis:** A strong primary care system should be the foundation for the entire health care system. This includes the right number of primary care providers, effective primary care models such as community health centers, and equitable, appropriate payment and reimbursement for primary care providers.

- **Affordable Coverage:** Most, but not all, people access their health care coverage through their work. To make sure access is good for everyone, Alaskan employers and individuals need to be able to purchase health care coverage at an affordable price.

- **Workforce Supports:** A strong primary care system needs a strong workforce. But in our current system, primary care providers make less money than specialists. Even when they'd prefer to practice primary care, students racking up huge educational loans choose better-paying specialty disciplines instead. Motivators such scholarship programs and loan repayment really help keep students in primary care. Alaska needs more of those programs.

- **Prevention Focused:** Taking good care of the body is key. To a point, we can prevent illness and disease by promoting awareness and active practice of good health and lifestyle choices. This education needs to be widely available because prevention and healthy lifestyle practices are learned behaviors and the place where they should primarily be learned - the home - is often not the place where they are well modeled.

- **Quality Focused:** Alaskans need to put a spotlight on quality. We need to assess quality through objective, transparent measures and publish outcomes and improvements.

- **Efficient and Appropriate Charges and Reimbursement:** We need to establish and maintain simple, transparent and honest processes for charging and paying for care, and focus on efficient, cost effective and accountable systems for payment.

- **Patient Engagement:** We must get Alaskans engaged in their care, and help them get to the very best status they can, regardless of their current health status. We can do this by promoting responsible patient self-management and partnership in care. Motivators could include incentives and rewards, such as reduced insurance premiums for healthy lifestyle choices. (On a side note, we should avoid punitive approaches because they don't work.)

- **Effective Models:** Models such as the patient centered medical home and other integrated models are proven to increase quality, contain or reduce costs and increase patient and provider satisfaction. Alaska needs these to become widespread.

- **Skin in the Game:** Every Alaskan, including the poor and underserved, needs to contribute to and share in the cost of their care in some way that is affordable and meaningful to them.

Governor, I know your goal is effective, efficient health care for current and future Alaskans. You have my support and that of countless others.

It's going to take considerable thought, effort and compromise to get there, and it will no doubt be painful. But we have no choice. Our kids are counting on us.

Sincerely,

Marilyn Kasmar

DEAR GOVERNOR:

WASHINGTON

RICHARD H. COOPER

Chief Executive Officer
The Everett Clinic

Dear Governor,

The Supreme Court decision to uphold the Affordable Care Act (ACA) has dominated the headlines. But now it is time to turn attention to the equally important issue of containing healthcare costs.

The ACA focuses primarily on providing more people with healthcare coverage and ways to pay for it. Now that more people are going to receive healthcare, the crucial issue is how to control costs.

The status quo is not sustainable. Healthcare costs are rising too fast and consuming an excessive amount of our economic output. Too much of the healthcare dollar is spent on expensive high-tech interventions. Not enough is spent to ensure people can

> Richard Cooper is the Chief Executive Officer of The Everett Clinic, which is independent medical group in Washington State. With more than 300 physicians at 9 locations throughout Snohomish County, the Clinic provides healthcare to approximately 295,000 patients each year, with expertise in more than 40 medical specialties.

DEAR GOVERNOR:

access basic primary care, which is more cost-effective.

The reform legislation provides an initial framework to transform healthcare. But it is too early tell what will actually be accomplished. Whether this legislation slows down the growth of healthcare costs, improves quality and increases access to care depends upon how the bill is implemented — and much of the implementation is left to the states.

Over the next few years, states will need to make important decisions about essential benefits, high-risk pools and healthcare exchanges. As a large purchaser of healthcare, our state needs innovative solutions that help contain costs. The state and taxpayers have a huge financial stake in policies that will reduce the cost of care while improving quality. If the state is willing to take the lead in adopting new approaches, change can be driven more easily throughout the marketplace.

The Everett Clinic adopted a goal of reducing costs by 25 percent over the next five years while improving quality. We have been working with a variety of partners including Boeing and the Center for Medicare and Medicaid Services to improve care delivery.

We believe our experiences point the way toward new approaches that our state, and other states, can replicate on a larger scale. Here is what we have learned so far:

- When primary care physicians and specialists regularly consult with each other and synchronize treatment, patient care is more cost-effective and achieves better outcomes. It makes sense to have the primary care doctor take the lead in planning a patient's care with specialists, hospitals, pharmacists and nursing homes. This kind of care coordination saves money by avoiding duplicate and unnecessary procedures and ensures that patients don't fall through the cracks.

- Paying to prevent illness rather than paying just to treat illness goes a long way to help control costs. Disease prevention saves lives and money, which is why Medicare will now pay for all proven preventive services without any cost sharing.

- Aggressively managing chronic diseases such as diabetes, asthma and heart disease ensures patients with on-going health problems receive the best preventive care possible. Disease management programs improve patients' quality of life, reduce hospitalizations and decrease the cost of care.

These three approaches – care coordination, prevention and disease management – can dramatically reduce one of the largest unnecessary costs in the system: the overuse of emergency rooms and hospitals.

Payment policies need to support and force change

These approaches to improve healthcare delivery can't be fully implemented unless healthcare payment policies are restructured. The top priority is to establish financial incentives for keeping patients healthy. This requires a huge shift in the traditional approach to medicine in the U.S., which historically has been disease-focused, not prevention-based.

Under the current fee-for-service payment model, providers see patients when they are already sick and receive a fee for each test or procedure. Not surprisingly, this payment system encourages overuse and drives up costs. Instead, providers should be rewarded for keeping patients healthy by interacting with them to manage and coordinate their care and ensure they follow recommended treatments.

For example, a patient with heart disease has weekly phone conversations with a nurse about how to effectively manage their diet, lifestyle and monitor their blood pressure. The on-going interaction avoids the need for more intense — and costly — interventions. Patients are pleased because they stay healthier and avoid unnecessary hospital stays.

The Boeing Intensive Outpatient Care Program is a specific example of how care coordination works and saves money. The Everett Clinic, Virginia Mason and Valley Medical Center worked with Boeing to help coordinate the care of employees who are high users of health services.

These complex patients were connected to a multidisciplinary care team that included a dedicated RN care manager and a supervising physician. A care plan was developed and executed through intensive in-person, phone and email communications. At the end of the program, the cost of care was reduced by 20 percent while improving care quality.

Increase use of evidence-based medicine

The use of evidence-based medicine – using proven treatments that result in the best patient outcomes – needs to be prioritized.

For example, better management of the use of expensive imaging tests such as MRIs and CT scans can save money. The Everett Clinic uses scientific evidence to develop specific guidelines for treating lower back pain, which results in fewer expensive imaging tests and lower costs, while maintaining high quality.

Generic prescribing is another proven way to reduce costs. Without sacrificing quality, The Everett Clinic has saved more than $88 million per year for patients, payors and taxpayers by prescribing generic drugs.

We employ our own pharmacists who independently examine evidence and make recommendations on prescribing methods. Pharmaceutical representatives and drug samples are not allowed in our facilities because prescribing decisions should be based on good science, not effective marketing.

Consumers need to take responsibility for their own health and seek value

Another key aspect of reducing healthcare costs is to reduce demand. We all need to take responsibility for managing our own health and staying well. We also need to become informed consumers when seeking medical care.

Consumers have unlimited opportunities to research a car before they purchase it, but little information is available about the experience of healthcare providers or the cost and effectiveness of various medical treatments. This information should be available and shared so consumers can make wise choices and informed decisions. As states establish healthcare exchanges, transparency should be a priority.

When it comes to healthcare, more is not necessarily better. This is especially true toward the end of life. Patients in the last few years of life account for more than 80 percent of healthcare costs. Yet, many of our patients tell us they do not want to spend their last days receiving intense medical care away from their homes and loved ones.

DEAR GOVERNOR:

Through a palliative care program, The Everett Clinic collaborates with hospice care to reach out to patients who are in the last one or two years of life. We work with patients and their families to offer care that reflects the patient's values and wishes. The goal is to increase satisfaction with end-of-life care and avoid unwanted hospitalizations and emergency room visits.

Healthcare reform must include a change in attitudes, not just laws

Devoting so much of our national spending to healthcare puts a huge financial strain on families, businesses, taxpayers and the entire economy. It also takes resources away from other priorities including job creation, education and other services.

The Affordable Care Act is an important first step to reform healthcare and increase access. Now efforts to contain healthcare costs become even more important. New approaches and partnerships are needed to ensure that healthcare is focused on value, not just volume — and on prevention, not just treatment. If healthcare costs can be successfully controlled, healthcare and insurance will become more affordable. When healthcare is affordable, more people will have the opportunity to access the care they need.

Sincerely,

Richard Cooper

DEAR GOVERNOR:

Acknowledgements

Building a book like this, a collection of diverse voices from leaders across the healthcare and policy spectrum, takes broad effort among many individuals. Without a commitment to deepening a public dialogue on healthcare from many, this book would not have come to pass.

First, thanks go to the many contributors to this project, those whose names appear on bylines in this book. There are also those whose names don't appear, but who were invaluable to the completion of the content here. Among those are folks like Eric Earling, Scott Forslund, Nicole Stewart, Holly Parsons, Misha Werschkul and April Zepeda.

The team here at Edmonds Publishing Group was also critical to the success of this effort. Particular thanks go to Jane Chemodanova and Mike Mestres for their hands on work. Kellee Bradley, Leo Cadiz, Nadica Kelley, Matt Wilcox and Nathaniel Currall also made important contributions to this project.

Finally, thanks go to my family. To Karianna, my wife, who understands the importance of seeding thoughtful discussion. To my son, Karsten, who has been patient with me as I worked on this book after reading only three books to him per night at bedtime. And, to my daughter, Annika, upon whose birth this project was inspired as I held her in the hospital on the first night of her life.

DEAR GOVERNOR:

About the Editor

DJ Wilson is the Publisher of the Edmonds Publishing Group, and hosts the State of Reform Health Policy Conferences. He has spent over 15 years in public policy, both in government and in the private sector.

DJ is also the President of Wilson Strategic Communications, one of the leading health care strategy and public affairs firms in the region.

DJ earned a Masters degree from the Johns Hopkins University, and his Bachelors degree from Gonzaga University. He has taught political science and economics courses at area colleges, including the University of Washington.

He lives with his wife and two children in Edmonds, Washington.

DEAR GOVERNOR:

About The State Of Reform

State of Reform is an organization committed to fostering dialogue and idea dissemination across the spectrum of health care today. To that end, in addition to this book, State of Reform takes on a number of initiatives.

State of Reform is a conference focused on bridging the gap between health care policy and political reality. Too often, those with good ideas for reforming health care don't have a solid grasp of how the legislative process works.

Those who understand politics don't always have a very deep grasp of the intricacies of the health care system. Our conferences – now held in four states – offer among the most sophisticated level of state-focused content of any health policy conference in the nation.

State of Reform – at www.stateofreform.com – is among the leading state health care news outlets in the country. With approximately 3000 unique visitors per week, the news site draws the attention of health care market executives and policy leaders alike.

State of Reform is an experiment in using social and digital media to seed thoughtful discussion. Through Twitter, Facebook and YouTube, State of Reform creates an online discussion space to connect with folks virtually. Through the monthly "5 Things

We're Watching" email newsletter, State of Reform tries to highlight key dynamics in the healthcare marketplace to an audience of over 20,000 readers.

Finally, State of Reform is a relationship – between speaker and listener, patient and provider, citizen and legislator. In a time of both antipathy and apathy towards solutions reliant or involving government, State of Reform is an experiment in republican democracy engaged in the most complicated public policy issue of the day: our health care.

Together, we're trying to improve the dialogue on health policy to support market and legislative outcomes of which we can all be proud.

DEAR GOVERNOR: